The Good Drinker

HOW I LEARNED TO LOVE DRINKING LESS

ADRIAN CHILES

P

PROFILE BOOKS

First published in Great Britain in 2022
and in this revised paperback edition in 2023
by Profile Books
29 Cloth Fair, Barbican, London EC1A 7JQ.
www.profilebooks.com

1 3 5 7 9 10 8 6 4 2

Typeset in Minion Pro and Blinker
to a design by Henry Iles.

A CIP catalogue record for this book is available from the
British Library.

ISBN 978-1788163606

eISBN 978-1782836179

Printed and bound by CPI Group (UK) Ltd, Croydon, CR0 4YY

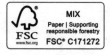

MIX
Paper | Supporting
responsible forestry
FSC
www.fsc.org
FSC® C171272

FOR KATH

Contents

Two important points

1

I was drinking an awful lot of alcohol. However, I wasn't waking up in shop doorways, wetting the bed, getting into fights or drinking Pernod in the morning. Therefore, I told myself, I obviously didn't have this 'disease' called 'alcoholism'. And, as I didn't have this 'disease', logically I was fine. I wasn't.

2

If I lined up all the drinks I'd drunk in a forty-year drinking career, stretching back to my mid-teens, that line would be around three miles long. This was quite a thought. More shocking than that, though, was the figure I got to when I considered how many of those drinks I could have done without. Or, put another away, how many of those had I really enjoyed, wanted or needed? I reckoned it was no more than a third of them. What a waste. Two miles of pointless drinks. This couldn't go on. All I had to do was find a way of enjoying the drinks I wanted, and not bother with the rest.

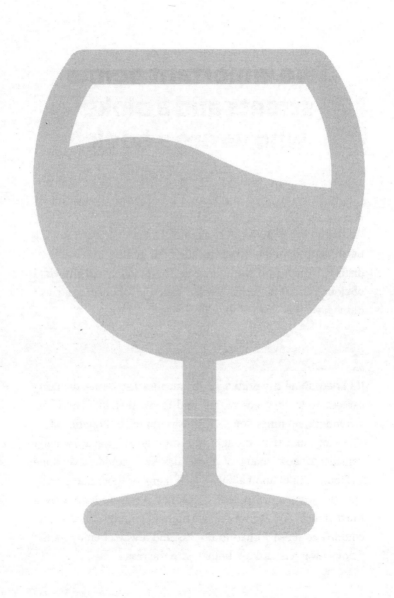

Two blokes in two streets and a bloke who wrote a book

Late one night in Manchester, I was walking back to my hotel after an evening out with some friends. A chap fell into step with me. He was plainly down on his luck, but decidedly chipper with it.

'I'm from Tipperary,' he told me. 'And I wonder if I could trouble you for some money, if you could spare some?'

I grunted something and we walked on for a moment before he added, 'And if you do give me any money, I make you this promise: I'll not be wasting it on food.'

I looked at him.

'No, I'll be spending it on booze!' he shouted in delight. 'Because I love booze.'

He won. I gave him a tenner.

I love booze too.
And I've learned to love it more by drinking less of it.

I was minding my own business down at the shops near where I live in West London when a bloke with a dog came up to me.

'There's a rumour you're off the booze,' he said.

'I've cut down a huge amount,' I replied.

'Oh, I see,' he said, smiling a knowing smile.

And off he went. I knew from the pitying look on his face exactly what he was thinking. He was thinking that I was in denial about my relationship with alcohol. In his view, there was no such as thing as cutting down. As I wasn't 'off the booze' completely, I plainly didn't have my drinking under control. I was kidding myself.

I get this a lot. It is annoying. It is widely held that the only realistic option available to heavy drinkers is to give up completely. This belief is so firmly held by many people that even if you do manage to convince them that you have genuinely moderated your drinking for good, they will simply conclude that you can't have had much of an alcohol problem in the first place. I get this a lot too. It is even more annoying.

There are certainly some problem drinkers for whom the only answer is to stop drinking completely. But I believe there are many more who don't seek help for their drinking precisely because they're frightened of being told that abstinence is their only option. This is a tragedy because, quite unable to countenance the prospect of life without alcohol, they just continue drinking as they were. Their consumption of alcohol won't be addressed, and they'll sink deeper into problem drinking territory and a level of dependence that means abstinence, in the end, really could be the only answer.

There's an awful lot of advice out there on how to stop drinking completely. In fact, there are so many moving and inspiring memoirs of journeys to sobriety that such books now have a genre to call their own: 'quit lit'. There's rather less lit available about drinking less alcohol.

Even Allen Carr's influential book, *The Easy Way To Control Alcohol*, isn't about moderation. It turns out to be about stopping drinking completely, but it's not until close to the end of the book that Carr comes clean about this:

Chronic drinkers would love to be able to control their intake, but have learned by hard experience that it has to be all or nothing. In between there are millions of drinkers who realise that they have a problem, but cannot face the prospect of life without alcohol; so they would love to be able to control their intake. If you are one of those drinkers, the title was deliberately designed to mislead you into believing that there is an easy way to be what AA [Alcoholics Anonymous] describes as a 'normal drinker'. I make no apologies for doing that. My sole objective was to prevent you going through further misery only to reach the inevitable conclusion that is has to be all or nothing.

It is to take nothing away from Carr's success in helping people stop drinking when I say that I disagree with him. For the millions of heavy drinkers who would like – or need – to control their intake, I don't believe it has to be 'all or nothing'. Furthermore, if those heavy drinkers believe it is so, then, as Carr tacitly acknowledges, many of them simply won't engage. If he'd called his book *The Easy Way to Stop Drinking*, he'd have sold a good deal fewer copies and, he insists:

The title I have used is truthful. There is an easy way to control your drinking. It happens to be the only way to control your drinking: TO BE COMPLETELY FREE.

To me, this is a bit like selling a book called *The Easy Way To Avoid Car Accidents*, in which the advice is not to get into a car.

In other words, Carr thinks that giving up completely is the easiest and only way to control your drinking. Obviously, I don't think abstinence is the only way. But, disingenuous as his book's title is, Carr does have a point: in some ways, stopping drinking completely is easier than drinking less. Giving up isn't easy, and moderating is really hard.

It can't be that hard though, if I've managed to pull it off.

I was drinking an awful lot; that much I appreciated. And writing this book has made me painfully aware of just how much my life revolved around alcohol. But now I do drink a lot less; I am living proof it is possible.

Furthermore, I've managed to do it without missing out on alcohol's benefits. I can honestly say that I now get greater enjoyment out of my drinking. Less has turned out to be more. Yes, I still have the odd mad night and sometimes drink too much over the course of a week, but the overall picture has changed.

In my experience, it can be done.

🍷 🥃 🍺

So, relax, this book definitely isn't a covert guide to knocking drinking on the head completely. Neither is it a classic self-help book. It might amount to the same thing, but it's really just a distillation, if you'll pardon the pun, of the many things I've learned about drinking less since I made a TV documentary on the subject* and started writing about it.

And what I've learned, you'll be shocked to read, is that it's complicated. Drinkers drink in different ways at different times for different reasons. So it follows that when it comes to

---

* The TV programme, made for BBC2, is called **Drinkers Like Me**. It is available from time to time on BBC iPlayer.

strategies for drinking less, there is no one strategy that is going to work for everyone. Far from it.

Actually, there's no one strategy that even works for me. Sometimes one thing works, sometimes it doesn't. And then it does again, once I go back to it, having tried something else which worked well, but then less well, and will probably work well again one day. And sometimes, if I'm honest, nothing works at all and I end up drinking too much over an evening, or a day, or a week. If that happens, I try not to be too hard on myself: a gentle word in my own ear is usually enough to have me reach into my moderation toolkit, find something that works, and pull things around again.

That's one advantage moderation has over abstinence: you don't need to feel like a complete failure if things go a bit wrong.

But it's undeniably one big, muddy muddle of an endeavour. It's not even clear what success or failure looks like. Moderation has no end point; no moment of jubilation or anniversary to celebrate. I was talking to the actress Finty Williams about this. She's had her difficulties with drinking and, happily, is now getting on famously having stopped altogether. During our conversation she told me that she was to spend that very evening going out to celebrate the, I think, second anniversary of her sobriety. While I was obviously delighted for her, it struck me that there is no equivalent for moderators: whoever heard of a group of friends gathering to celebrate a year of moderation? For a start, how much should you drink? What if it got rowdy and the people at the next table asked what you were celebrating? I can't think of anything you could say that wouldn't sound ridiculous. On the other hand, why not? It might encourage more people to give moderation a whirl.

An acquaintance of mine, Laura Willoughby, puts it rather nicely. Laura founded Club Soda, an organisation which promotes the radical notion that a social life without any, or much, alcohol is actually possible.

People who are moderating tend not to shout about it, she says. *Because moderation is always a work in progress. It's never finished. There is no end point ...*

She's right; there is no end point. There is, however, a starting point and, even if you've only read this far, it's possible you're at that starting line now. And if you're reading this with a drink in your hand, so be it. Don't panic. It doesn't have to be your last.

My starting point

A few years ago, I arrived in Manchester one Sunday evening on a train from Euston. I was in a bit of a grump. Though I lived in London, my work in the early part of the week involved broadcasting from the BBC in Salford. This journey always felt like a bit of a slog. Sunday evenings are a bad time to travel; the trains are packed, and everyone's pissed off because the weekend's over. On this particular Sunday, back at home, I'd had a glass or two of wine at lunch, and a pint of lager with a curry at a restaurant near Euston. I'd dozed off on the train. Walking down the big ramp out of Piccadilly I looked up to see a huge poster paid for by Alcoholics Anonymous. It featured a park bench, covered in snow. Above it were the words, YOU DON'T HAVE TO LIVE HERE TO CALL US.

Hmm. It was 9.30pm and I was just contemplating a couple of drinks in the bar at the hotel I stay in, next to the station. And, sure enough, I bumped into a guy I knew and drank some Guinness with him.

I kept thinking about that poster. I knew the recommended maximum intake for men and women was 14 units of alcohol a week. That day my two glasses of wine would have come to 5 units, and the pint at Euston and two Guinnesses in the hotel were another 7. So that's 12 units in one day; nearly my whole recommended weekly limit. And here's the thing: this wasn't even really *drinking* in my book. It was just what I drank if I wasn't really drinking. It was my baseline level of drinking; my default drinking position.

And then I went to bed, already looking forward to the following evening when once again I would have a couple of drinks in the bar followed by a couple of glasses of wine with dinner (around 9 units). Then, the following evening when I got back home to London, I would doubtless meet my mate for a couple of pints when he finished work (another 5 units at least). So I'd be at least 50 per cent above my weekly limit by Tuesday evening.

The poster now really made sense. It wasn't that I felt I needed to call Alcoholics Anonymous there and then, but I did take the point that just because I was sleeping in room 432 of the Malmaison Hotel, rather than on a park bench, that didn't mean I had no issue with alcohol.

🍷 🍺 🥛

I started drinking in my teens, very enthusiastically. I carried on in my twenties, seeing no reason to stop. In my thirties I had small children but still spent lots of time in pubs, and I drank at home too. By my forties I was famous and successful and doing a lot of socialising which always, but always, involved drinking. Going into my fifties it struck me that I'd drunk more in my forties than in my thirties, when I'd drunk more than I had in my twenties and my teens.

I suspected this couldn't be good, but apart from being a bit overweight there were no obvious issues. I always did plenty of exercise, and lost weight by changing the food I ate. I didn't do much drinking during the day and I wasn't one for late nights. I hardly got hangovers and rarely got what you might call drunk. I didn't get into fights or rows and if I did anything daft I couldn't blame alcohol for it, because I would most likely have done the same thing sober.

On the face of it there was no need to worry, but I've always had a gift for finding things to worry about and my drinking was no exception. I had dinner with a close friend, the comedian and writer Frank Skinner. Frank used to be, in his words, a Pernod-in-the-morning type drinker. His drinking nearly finished him off, but he gave it up and hasn't touched a drop now for many decades, during which time his career has gone from strength to strength.

Sitting in this restaurant, he was saying, not for the first time, how he envied me what he called my level of drinking – essentially my ability to drink sociably without ending up falling asleep in a skip. I nodded, but I knew it wasn't quite as simple as that. Looking to illustrate this point I came up with a hypothetical:

You know how sociable I am? Well, if there was a gathering over the road from here this evening, of a hundred friends and acquaintances who I really liked, I'd be looking forward to the event very much. But if, for whatever reason, I couldn't drink, I'd be pretty much dreading it.

Frank was somewhat horrified and, on reflection, I was too. Really, what difference would it possibly make if I couldn't drink? My friends' delightful company is great; that's why we're friends. Why would I need drink inside me to enjoy it?

The question niggled away. Around this time, I was talking to a woman called Fiona at a Christmas gathering of some old school friends. She was telling me how much she liked, or perhaps needed, a glass of wine every night. I asked her how she'd feel if she was told, for health reasons, that she wasn't allowed to drink anymore. She had a little think and said, bluntly enough, 'I'd shit myself.'

I found this shocking, not least because I had to admit I felt the same way. I, like her, would feel nothing less than fear if I was told I had to live my life without alcohol.

Yet, according to what it is generally understood to be an alcoholic, I wasn't one. I'd been led to believe that an alcoholic was someone who, upon having one drink, was quite unable to stop until they collapsed in a gutter somewhere. It was a genetic thing apparently. They were born that way. They drank in the morning, they wet the bed, they were incapable of lucid conversation, they looked funny, they smelt funny, they were obviously in poor health and they were frequent visitors to A&E.

I was none of these things, so surely had nothing to worry about; I was in the clear. I could carry on drinking as deeply as I saw fit.

🍷🥃🍺

My dad, in his view, is none of these things either. As a pot calls a kettle black, I frequently bend his ear about drinking. Half his life ago he had to have a heart bypass operation, having developed angina. I recall him relating the conversation he'd had with the cardiologist about his alcohol intake. 'I told him I drank about a bottle of wine a day, and a bottle of whisky a week,' my dad said. Or at least that's what he told me he'd told him. He claimed the cardiologist batted not an eyelid at this revelation, which my dad took to mean that this doctor considered such an intake perfectly normal.

More than three decades on, I popped in to see Dad one day. He asked me what I had coming up at work. I told him I was trying to get a television documentary made about alcohol dependence. He pulled a face to indicate what an unsavoury business he considered such a thing to be. This of course led to something of an argument, during the course of which he said, 'I'm not an alcoholic. That kind of drinking's all about running around at night shouting and making a mess. I'm nothing like that.'

I looked at the large glass of wine in his hand, and then at the clock. It was 12.20 on a Thursday lunchtime.

'So if you're nothing like that,' I asked. 'What are you like?'

'I'm a moderate drinker,' he declared, with some confidence. We continued bickering on this theme for a bit longer before we both shrugged and moved on.

The trouble is that everyone's got a different idea of what moderate drinking looks like. To my dad, a bottle of wine a day and a bottle of spirits a week had for a long time been his idea of moderate. And, according to him anyway, only a couple of the countless doctors who'd kept him alive into his eighties had ever contested the point. So, for him, as long as he isn't resembling the caricature of the alcoholic he carries in his head, he doesn't have a problem.

And who could blame him for taking that view? Until recently, it's exactly the view I'd taken. Because all drinkers – and this is the vast majority of us – who aren't the alcoholic of caricature take great comfort from that and award ourselves free passes to carry on boozing with impunity. You are either An Alcoholic, or you're not. Simple. It's probably something you're born with. So hard luck if you've got it; lucky you if you haven't.

But how could I possibly convince myself I didn't have some kind of serious dependence on alcohol when I couldn't remember the last time I'd gone a day without it; when I was drinking more with each year that passed and, hell, I couldn't even fancy an evening with all my nearest and dearest friends if there wasn't drink involved?

It's next to impossible to get a television programme commissioned at the best of times, but *Drinkers Like Me* proved to be particularly difficult to get away. Every other documentary ever made about drinking seemed to feature drinkers who all of us could be clear were alcoholics. Blue lights flashed, much vomit was in evidence, and lives were devastated. There was drama at every turn. In the cynical parlance of my industry, there were money shots galore.

I understood why this worked for television, and also why it is important that these awful stories were told. But that doesn't alter the fact that drinkers like these were, are, and hopefully always will be, in a tiny minority. By focusing only on them, the whole drinking picture had been gravely distorted. The many dangerously heavy drinkers, drinkers like me, never got any coverage.

The commissioners took this point but kept worrying about what exactly we would point the camera at for our film. Me drinking too much, but behaving quite sensibly and without any drama, would unquestionably be a rather dull watch. But I kept hammering on that this was the very reason that the story, about the dangers of being one of the millions of 'drinkers like me', never got told.

Eventually the commissioners relented, and we got the green light. And now it was my turn to worry about what on earth we were going to film; I actually got concerned that I wasn't a big enough drinker to justify making the documentary. I needn't have worried. Two things happened early on in production, both on camera, that changed everything for me.

The first filming we did was on a Saturday, around a football match between my team, West Brom, and Liverpool. It was a pretty standard Saturday for me: in the pub with mates before an early kick-off, back home to London in the afternoon for a friend's fortieth birthday in the evening, and I was tucked up in bed by 1am. Come Sunday morning the crew turned up at my place to film me working out how much I'd drunk the day before. I'd always resisted doing these sums. The truth is that it took getting a television documentary commissioned for me to box myself into a corner where I just had to do it.

I'd drunk four pints of Guinness in the pub before the game. That's on the high side for me ahead of a match, but by no means unheard of. As it was an early kick-off, I was away from the ground by 2.30. I then didn't drink anything until I was back in London, in the East End, for the birthday party. I started off with a couple of thirst-quenching beers, followed by the obligatory glass of champagne. Then it was on to several glasses of red wine during dinner and then another pint of lager, because someone handed me one and I was thirsty.

That lot totted up to 38 units of alcohol. It's generally thought that if you're drinking more than 14 units a week you will start damaging your health. So, on a pretty unexceptional Saturday for me, during which I never felt remotely drunk, I'd put away more than two and a half times what is considered to be safe to drink in a whole week. And it didn't take me long to calculate that over the course of my average week I was drinking getting on for 100 units of alcohol. Sobering news.

And there was more to come. A few days later I was lying face down on a treatment table in a Harley Street clinic awaiting a liver scan. 'Turn over,' sighed the hepatologist. 'Your liver's at the front.' Who knew? I turned onto my back for him to splurge a little gel on me and set about scanning. As he did so, he muttered darkly something about fat and the difficulty of getting a reading, but I remained unconcerned. Why, only a few weeks before, I'd had some blood tests at my GP which had turned up nothing of interest.

He disappeared back to his office where, gel wiped off and shirt back on, I found him engrossed in his computer screen. The next few minutes are a bit of a blur. He said something about mild cirrhosis and a fatty liver and stuff like that. The one thing I remember clearly was him saying, firmly and with neither compassion nor criticism, 'Something's got to change; you can't go on like this.'

I also recall asking him, rather desperately, if he didn't enjoy a drink. He told me he liked a Guinness 'every now and then, every couple of weeks perhaps'. I judged him to be a most eccentric fellow. Dazed, I made my way to the lift, followed by a camera. This was bad news indeed.

The better news is that I sit here, a couple of years on, having heeded that doctor's advice. Something did change; I didn't go on the way I had been. I still enjoy drinking, but I've found a way of drinking a great deal less. I used to drink between 50 and 100 units a week; these days I'm down to something between 10 and 30. I'm not sure whether this counts as a rather modest achievement or a bit of a triumph. Either way, this book's about how I managed to change my ways and drink a great deal less.

I've no idea if how I've achieved this is relevant to you, or someone you know, but hopefully there's something useful in here for anyone who drinks too much and wants to drink less, but without giving up completely.

Looking back

I'm not a fan of looking back in the way a lot of therapy demands. The way I see it, therapy should help you do three things:

1 See what you are really like, how you think and how you behave.

2 Work out why it is that you are the way you are.

3 Establish how you might go about changing the things about yourself that need changing.

I've always thought that point 1 is harder than you think and point 3 is really hard full stop. This being the case, why get too bogged down on point 2?

To my mind, the conclusions reached often amount to not much more than speculation. Yes, a girl might have said something nasty to me during a game of kiss chase in a primary school playground in 1974, but I really didn't think it was right or fair to pin a lifetime's hang-ups on that particular girl in that particular playtime.*

However, when it came to writing about how I've managed to drink less, it seemed reasonable to have a look back at my life to examine how it was that I came to be drinking quite so much. I had no intention of writing a memoir, not least because I couldn't imagine anyone wanting to read it. Tellingly though, I found I couldn't reflect on my drinking life without talking about the rest of my life because, depressingly, it turns out the two are tightly intertwined.

If you see your life as a rotating circle, you should find yourself at its centre. For sure, you'll often be pulled and pushed and buffeted away from the hub of your wheel, but the centre is where you belong. The feeling I get is that for the first two-thirds of my life it was not me in the middle, but alcohol. There it has been, sitting at the centre of my wheel, while around it I have revolved. This makes me very sad. No serious harm done perhaps; I've done well for myself and mustn't grumble, but it shouldn't have been this way.

For the last third of my life (assuming I live past the age of seventy-five), alcohol can have its place, but no longer will it be at the centre of my wheel.

---

* She told me the reason that all the girls chased me, rather than anyone else, wasn't because they wanted to kiss me. It was because I was the only boy slow enough for them to catch. Hurtful.

Early years

My Uncle Gerald, one of my dad's oldest friends, came around every Thursday evening to pick my dad up to go to the pub for a couple of pints. They were old mates, which was good, and their drinking beer together was apparently both a cause and effect of that, so beer was good too.

My mum barely drank, bar a daily shot of šljivovica, Croatian plum brandy so strong that it was almost beyond even my dad's tolerance. He called it U-boat fuel. My mum said it was good for you because it killed all germs. So strong stuff seemed to be good too.

My grandad used to pick me up every other Saturday at midday to take me to West Bromwich Albion's home games. On the way we'd always stop at the same chip shop in Smethwick where my grandad would buy me chicken and chips with curry sauce poured over the top. I'd sit with it wrapped up on my knees for the rest of the short journey. The aroma of the food, scented with the chip paper, made my mouth water. My mouth is watering now. We'd park behind the supporters' club, on the car park facing the back of the Rainbow Stand, where our seats were. Kick-off would still be more than two hours away. My grandad would go off and meet his old friend Frank in the supporters' club bar. I'd remain in the passenger seat, retrieve the cutlery my nan had left for me in the glove box and set about demolishing the chicken and chips with curry sauce poured over the top.

I'd then spend the next couple of hours sitting in the car listening to the build-up to the match on local radio. I'd try to concentrate on doing some homework, but I was usually too absorbed watching all the people and cars crowding into view through the windscreen. I've rarely in my life known such a wonderful combination of excitement, fascination and sheer unalloyed pleasure.

Grandad would emerge from the supporters' club bar at exactly 2.40pm to take me into the ground, bringing reliably the best couple of hours of my week to an end (the match itself was often less enjoyable). I'll never stop being grateful to my grandad for those two hours of car-bound bliss. And it all happened in order for him to enjoy a couple of pints with his mate Frank. They were happy. I was happy. And it was beer that made it all possible. Beer was good.

I've occasionally been asked why it is that I need to go for a drink before watching the Albion play. And I've always answered with something lame, along the lines of, 'You wanna try watching us sober...' etc. etc. It was only during the COVID pandemic, having been forced to take a break from my live Albion-watching, that I asked myself the same question. Where does this urge come from? I've raced off to games hours early to give me a chance to drink a lot of beer in a relatively short time. Every now and again, with delicious symmetry, I have a beer with Richard, grandson of none other than my grandad's drinking mate Frank. Yes, the craic with my Albion mates is good, usually. Sometimes it isn't. Occasionally it's all rather boring. But I always make the effort. Why? Well, I blame my grandad.

This is something he would take great exception to. He wasn't even a big drinker; at home he'd have the odd beer in a pint glass with a handle but that was about it. Strange, then, that the only other regular outing I'd have with him also involved drinking. On a Sunday lunchtime he and my nan would drive me, my brother and their Yorkshire Terrier, Mandy, off to a pub called The Reindeer on the road to Worcester. This place was chosen because it had a goat tied up out the back. 'Let's go and see the nanny goat,' trilled my nan as we headed off there.

On arrival we'd dutifully stand and stare at the nanny goat while Mandy yapped away in the car. The nanny goat would stare back. I don't recall either my brother or me expressing any particular interest in goats. But we didn't mind because we loved being with our grandparents. Although, once there, we weren't really with them for long, as Nan and Grandad would go into the pub leaving the two of us in the car with Mandy. One of them would emerge briefly with pop and crisps, before disappearing again. But everyone was happy. Drinking was nice, drinking was good.

My early life afforded me hardly any bad alcohol-related experiences. We were on a family holiday once, walking around some foreign city, when we turned a corner to be confronted by an obviously drunk homeless bloke. The poor man was roaring in distress, anger, confusion, or some combination of the three. This was shocking to me.

The only person I ever recall seeing properly drunk at our house was Colin, husband of one of my mum's friends. His skin was a strange, leathery reddish-brown. At a Sunday afternoon gathering of some sort at our house I saw him lean on one of my dad's hi-fi speakers. Either Colin or the loudspeaker or both toppled over. This was shocking too.

'He's an alcoholic,' my dad explained later.

'What's that?'

'It's someone who just can't stop drinking.'

Before long, Colin was dead. He must have been in his forties, younger than I am now. But this didn't put me off alcohol, or even really alert me to the dangers of it. After all, Colin had this thing called alcoholism, which was just his bad luck, like having a bad back or a dodgy ticker.

So it was that the only two bad, alcohol-related experiences of my boyhood featured alcoholics of caricature.

Elsewhere, drinking-wise, it was all good.

Perhaps my drinking life would have been different if it had been otherwise.

🍷 🥛 🍺

I remember my own first drink very clearly. I was thirteen years old and we were at a family party somewhere in Birmingham. My cousin Katie and I were in the back garden standing by a trestle table. I picked up a glass of something fizzy which was almost as sweet as squash. I later found out it was called cider. It gave me a thrilling energy with which to tear around the house and garden, laughing and shouting. I felt good all over. It was real fun. I don't think anything especially dramatic happened, but perhaps it did because on the way home my dad had cause to say to me, 'You have to be careful with cider. I remember when I was a kid, beer tasted awful, but cider was different. Cider was just like pop.'

The only other pre-pubescent drinking I recall was over Sunday lunch. Sometimes the wine would be in a brown bottle with the word 'Oktober' on the label. I discovered this wine was nice and sweet, like the cider, so I enjoyed a bit of that. It didn't seem to affect me much. My dad always drank a lot; my mum less so. But drinking was the norm in our house.

When I was fourteen I went on school exchange to Germany. I was paired up with a lad who I'll call Siegfried, with whom I had nothing in common. This was entirely my own fault because at the time I filled in the form about my interests, I had just decided to take up chess. I duly declared chess to be my main interest in life. It wasn't. My main interests were football, music and the unrequited adoration of a succession of girls. Chess was only on that list for about four days, before I realised that I neither understood nor enjoyed it. I gave it up. By then, though, the wheels of the penfriend selection machine were turning. It needed no particularly great application of Teutonic logic for me to be paired up with a keen member of the German school's chess club.

Poor Siegfried looked every inch the junior chess enthusiast. He wore the kind of glasses that make your eyes look bigger. I too had started to wear glasses, for short sight, so I suppose we did have specs in common, but that was it.

The whole trip got off to an appalling start the day before it began. I got home from school and sensed straight away that something wasn't right, in a kind of not-quite-rightness I hadn't come across before. Soon my dad was telling me that my grandmother in Croatia was gravely ill. Baka, as I called her, had had a stroke in her flat in Zagreb. My mum was speaking urgently to her sister on the phone. I was close to my Baka; she spent every Christmas with us. I really didn't want to go on the stupid German exchange. I was terribly upset and anxious and, anyway, the correspondence between us had already strongly suggested that Siegfried wasn't my type.

But Mum and Dad decided I should go. I fervently wished they hadn't. I'd never been so miserable in all my life. Come to think of it, I've not been so miserable since. Never have two weeks passed so slowly for anyone ever. The school was in a small town near Stuttgart. Not only did I get on with Siegfried every bit as badly as I'd feared, he didn't seem to be friends with any of his classmates on the exchange. He kept saying he was friends with a lad who was partnered with a friend of mine called Russell. I thought this would mean I could at least hang out with Russell a bit, but Russell told me that this lad didn't want anything to do with Siegfried.

I looked longingly at my fellow schoolmates all having wonderful times with their new friends. The German girls were conspicuously beautiful and plainly uninterested in either me or my fellow spectacle wearer. We shambled wordlessly home. To Siegfried's understandable bafflement I refused all his offers of a game of chess. Eventually I relented just to show him how clueless I was, which didn't take long. No more chess was played.

To make matters even worse, a friend from home sent me a press cutting about Bryan Robson, my team's best player, being sold to Manchester United. If it was possible to die of sheer dismay, this would have been the moment I drew my last breath.

I was so homesick it physically hurt. A couple of days after I arrived, my mum called. She said: 'The situation in Zagreb is unchanged, and we're going there tomorrow.' The situation in Zagreb is unchanged? Since when did my Mum talk like that? She was obviously parroting a line my dad had given her, or she'd heard on the news. I knew then that my Baka had died. I sank still lower. Siegfried's mother was a lovely woman who could see how miserable I was. The poor thing tried everything to cheer me up, without success.

I have scant memory of any of the excursions our exchange group were taken on, bar one. In the second week we went on a tour of the town's brewery. I moped around, disliking the smell of the place, looking on without interest as we were shown how beer was made. Unaccountably, at the conclusion of the tour this group of fourteen- and fifteen-year-olds were sat down at long tables and given rather strong lager to drink. I didn't much enjoy it but, within a matter of minutes of it coursing through my veins, I was going through some kind of emotional transformation. It felt so good. In an instant the last few days we had left on the exchange went from feeling like an eternity to something wispy and insignificant and even possibly enjoyable. I laughed and joked with my friends and even fancied I spotted a girl called Claudia looking at me. And I became overwhelmed with sorrow for Siegfried who couldn't face more than a mouthful of beer but, with unbearable sweetness, was plainly delighted to see me smiling for once. Waves of wellbeing felt like they were crashing over me.

It's only now, writing this, that I see how significant that afternoon was in my whole drinking story. It came at a traumatic moment in a critically formative phase of my life. I'd never had to deal with the death of a loved one before. I was going through shock, bewilderment, fear, loneliness and terrible, gut-wrenching homesickness. I was in pain. But one draught of this strange brew took that pain away. In the matter of a few minutes my whole world had been reframed. It was magical. The psychological die was cast.

Even if this episode had ended with me spewing up everywhere, or waking up with a throbbing headache, I doubt it would have made any difference. The relief it gave me was so intense that I'm sure I would have felt illness a price worth paying. As it was, I experienced no ill effects at all. The power of alcohol had been cast in a decidedly favourable light.

🍷🥛🍺

Having discovered the benefits of intoxication it seemed like common sense to dabble in it some more. And, with growing excitement, dabble I did. I pilfered cans of lager, bottles of wine and tots of spirits from my dad's stash. These I'd drink with a mate or two when my parents were out, or at someone else's house, or in a field, outside a school disco, at a party, or outside a party if there was no booze allowed. On one occasion my friend Martyn hatched a cunning plan which involved acquiring some cans from somewhere, bidding his parents goodbye as we left the house, and turning right, right and right again down the road to the cemetery which ran past the bottom of his garden. Then we clambered over the fence across the lawn and into his dad's shed. Here we spent a very pleasant, if chilly, few hours drinking Banks's Bitter, smoking roll-ups and listening to *The Friday Rock Show* on Radio One.

I was fifteen when I first got properly drunk. I had a small part in the school production of *Oliver!*. I was infatuated with one of the flower girls, Helen, who was in the year above me and wore a lot of make-up. My friend Jamie had a bigger part in the show. He played Mr Sowerberry and was in love with Nancy, who was played by Angela, the school beauty. She too was in the year above us, and entirely beyond the reach of any boy anywhere as far as either of us could discern.

Jamie's older brother was prevailed upon to get us some alcohol for the party after the last show. He bought an extra-large bottle of wine. I felt its weight, appreciatively.

'Soave,' I read from the bottle.

'Good with fish,' said Jamie.

'How do you know?'

'Think I remember my dad saying something about it.'

We carried it up to the school in the bag I used for my newspaper round and hid it beneath a temporary classroom.

As soon as the curtain came down, the two of us raced outside and necked the Soave straight out of the bottle. What happened next remains uncertain, shrouded in a cloud of shame and embarrassment. All I can remember for sure is that I ended up outside with Helen, watching adoringly as she swigged out of our bottle. I could hold back my ardour for not a moment longer and declared undying love for her. She laughed at me. Laughed! And walked away.

Disconsolate I bumbled off to the buffet laid on in the sixth-form common room where I comfort-ate several slices of pizza topped with sardines. It brought me no comfort. I was in an ecstasy of humiliation and misery. There was no sign of Jamie, so I went to see if he was outside with our Soave stash. He wasn't. Here, at the scene of my recent rejection, I made my one and only good decision of the evening: I decided not to finish the wine. Heartbreakingly, Helen's lipstick was still on the neck of the bottle.

A study in disappointment, I shambled away in the direction of Jamie's house where I was due to sleep over. Before I was out of the school gates, I had a tap on the shoulder. It was Angela. 'Do you know where Jamie is?' she asked.

My mouth opened and closed but nothing came out. I shook my head.

'Oh no,' she moaned to a friend next to her. 'I think he's gone. I really like Jamie. He's so sweet.'

They ran off back to the party, giggling.

Somehow, I got back to Jamie's house where he was sitting in the kitchen with his parents. 'She loves you,' I shouted. 'Angela loves you!' I'd all but forgotten my own disaster, such was my joy at my friend's good fortune. He was as delighted as his mum and dad were concerned at the sight of these two teenagers pissed out of their silly heads. We were ushered off to bed. I was put in Jamie's sister's room, as she was away at university.

I awoke an hour or two later to find myself vomiting sardine pizza and Soave all over myself, the bed and the carpet. It was a gruesome scene. Jamie's parents got me onto the floor of his bedroom, threw a duvet over me, and commenced the clean-up operation. For the second time in one evening I'd comprehensively humiliated myself. At least there was a certain pleasing symmetry to be found woven through the carnage: wine, thought to be good with fish, bought by Jamie's brother, mixed with fish and vomited all over their sister's bedroom.

In the morning, beside myself with remorse, I apologised to everyone. They were really very good about it. Jamie put 'Fool If You Think It's Over' by Chris Rea on the record player.

'This is for you,' he said. 'Because it's not over with you and Helen.'

He was wrong there. It was not only over; it had never happened in the first place. Eventually I left and walked home. I still felt terrible. I'd made a right dick of myself. It had been a night of shame. And yet, absurdly, I felt as much pride as shame, a sense of achievement even. I'd got properly pissed and puked everywhere. I couldn't wait for word to get out about this triumph. I had turned the corner into manhood.

🍷🥃🍺

What could have been different, I wonder? What might have happened to choke off this nascent love of alcohol; this dependence, addiction – call it what you will – before it took root?

As well as what I experienced amongst my family and friends, the cultural ubiquity of alcohol must have had an influence on me. Many experts in the field are clear that seeds of interest in alcohol are sown in young minds in all sorts of ways, such as advertising and other stuff you see on TV. So, in terms of legislative intervention, I suppose a ban on alcohol advertising before the watershed might have been a help, although drinking was all around me anyway.

My relationship with alcohol is similar to the one I have with my football team. I've spent a lot of time exploring the nature of the psychological hold West Bromwich Albion have over me. A cognitive anthropologist I came across, Dr Martha Newson, had spent time studying what on earth goes on between the ears of football fanatics like me. In her field, if you're exceptionally passionate and loyal to something you are said to be fused with it. Yes, hands up, I'm fused with West Brom. Good word for it, that: fused. And it's just as good a word to describe my relationship with alcohol. I don't know how old I was when a psychologist might have judged me to be clinically fused with booze, but the process was certainly well underway before I'd started shaving.

What could have stopped this fusion from taking place? I suppose the easiest thing would have been if I'd swallowed that cider at my cousin's party, hated the taste of it, spat it out or, even better, spewed it up. Might that have killed it off at birth? Or what about if the giddy time I was having that night had led to a stumble over my nan's leg, a cracked head and a trip to hospital for the pair of us? I doubt even that would have made a difference because by then, losing copious amounts of blood or not, I'd already experienced that gorgeous giddiness. Perhaps there was already no going back.

It might have helped if my dad had said something other than the thing about cider being dangerously nice. As it was, he inadvertently planted the idea that cider was two things sure to pique the interest of any teenager: dangerous and nice. Cider, I'd learned, was dangerously pleasurable – and pleasurably dangerous. Noted.

How else could he have put it?

'You looked stupid, running around giggling like that.'

'Alcohol's full of sugar; it'll make you fat.'

Or: 'You had a good time, didn't you? You do know you'd have had just as good a time if you hadn't drunk that cider?'

I blame him not a jot for not saying any of these things, by the way. Not least because I doubt they'd have made any difference; I was already on my way.

The German brewery trip was a game changer – for good in the short-term but unquestionably for ill in the long run. It reframed the misery of my situation so dramatically that I'll always be grateful for what alcohol did for me that day. And for that reason, paradoxically, try as I might, I can't bring myself to wish it had never happened.

Neither can I feel anything but warm memories for the evening Martyn and I spent in his dad's shed. But with the Oliver-Helen-Soave-sardine-sickness debacle, it gets more interesting. What if, instead of laughing at my declaration of love, Helen had responded in kind. 'I think you're wonderful too, Adrian. Please will you kiss me?' And what if then, as my heart swelled, so did a wave of nausea, causing me to discharge a bellyful of Soave everywhere, and Helen to walk away in disgust? Seriously, I may never have forgiven alcohol for that; the course of my drinking life might have been changed forever.

Teenage drinks scorecard

● CONSUMPTION

Difficult to say. The most at one sitting would have been possibly **7 units**. Averaged out, my weekly intake would have been negligible.

● BORING BITS

There weren't any.

● PROPORTION OF DRINKS WANTED/NEEDED/ENJOYED

100 per cent.

What qualifies me to write this book

Not a lot, would be one answer, I suppose. I don't have much in the way of science qualifications. C grades in O level physics and chemistry, achieved in the summer of 1983, are the beginning and end of it.

Nor do I have a dramatic tale to tell of drinking myself to the very edge of sanity before reining it in, or giving up, in the nick of time. No, my drinking story is more mundane. But this is the key point: most dangerous drinking stories are mundane. The very mundanity of drinking stories like mine is the most dangerous thing about them. We go way under the radar, yet most cases of health blighted by heavy drinking are among drinkers like me. There's generally very little drama in our drinking stories, until perhaps the day a doctor looks up and says we're pickled.

It's not that we're the most likely to run into medical problems. That honour goes to the most prodigious of heavy drinkers, the 'alcoholics' of caricature. They account for roughly five per cent of drinkers. However, it's in the next bracket, where I was, that most harm is to be found, basically because there are so many more of us; about a quarter of all drinkers, in fact. These are – or were – my people. Boringly, relentlessly, mundanely putting lots of it away, often without anyone, least of all ourselves, realising the harm we are doing.

Sparing my blushes, I now consider myself a bona fide expert in this level of drinking. Ever since I made *Drinkers Like Me*, I've unwittingly found myself to be a kind of one-man focus group, counsellor, researcher and confessor, to, about and for drinkers, ex-drinkers, teetotallers and families of drinkers everywhere.

Wherever I go, indoors, outdoors, eating, drinking, walking or whatever, people come up to me and talk with disarming frankness about their drinking. They're generally neither proud nor ashamed, merely curious and keen to talk to a kindred spirit. I seem to have made myself relatable to people across the whole spectrum of alcohol use, misuse and non-use. Having publicly acknowledged that I had some kind of problem, I seem to be in good odour with people whom you might loosely label the anti-alcohol lobby. This includes recovering alcoholics, obviously, and anyone whose life has really been blighted by booze. It also includes many healthcare professionals – family doctors, counsellors, psychologists, psychiatrists and very many hepatologists – liver specialists.

On the other hand, because I also made clear in the programme how much I enjoyed drinking, and would continue to do so, enthusiastic drinkers of all kinds throw their arms around me, physically and metaphorically. A good example: I was watching West Brom play at Swansea City. During the interval I needed to use the gents, but to avoid the half-time crush I waited until the second half had started. Standing there, doing what I'd gone in for, a young man recognised me. He had a cigarette in his mouth and was holding a full pint of beer. Using his free hand he was just zipping up. He came in for a big, smoky, beery hug even though I was still doing my business.

'I fucking love you, Ade,' he said, clinging onto me like a baby koala. 'I love the Albion like you do, and I really fucking loved that drinking programme you did. Fucking brilliant,' he concluded.

I'm far too shallow to be anything but pathetically grateful for any kind of affirmation. But you have to wonder, that if this chap loved our team so much, why was he drinking and smoking in the gents when he could have been in his seat watching the match? And if he thought the drinking programme was so great, how come he was pissed out of his head now?

This kind of thing happens a lot.

It doesn't make sense, but an awful lot of stuff around drinking doesn't make sense. Outside the away end at Millwall's ground the other day, a grizzled West Brom fan about my age collared me.

'Loved your drinking show; I drank like you,' he told me, and went on to explain how drinking had ruined his health so he'd had to pack it in.

'Did you feel better for it?' I asked.

'Yes.'

'Oh great, so you still not drinking?'

'Nah, back on it now, ain't I? You gotta, aintcha?'

And into the ground we went. We lost 2-0, by the way.

If I'd carried a tape recorder with me at all times, I could fill a book with stuff complete strangers have told me. Shortly after the programme was broadcast, at another West Brom away game – at Birmingham City on a Friday night, since you ask – I got a tap on my shoulder during the half-time break. A vast bloke with tattoos and a shaven head had clambered across many seats to ask for my view on a medical matter.

'I drink sixty pints of lager a week. Do you think that's too much?' he demanded.

Absurdly, I found myself adopting the kindly, non-judgemental tone of a concerned GP.

'Well,' I said. 'You could consider cutting down a little bit, I suppose?'

He looked like he wanted something more definite than that, so, using what I'd recently learned about the lore of 'mindful' drinking (more on which later), I tried a different tack.

'Listen, from what I know, that's an awful lot more to drink than is good for you and any doctor ought to tell you that. But I'm not a doctor so what I'd say to you is: if you're drinking all those sixty pints of lager and really loving the bones of every single one of them, then who is anyone to tell you not to do it? But honestly, are you actually enjoying every drop of all that beer?'

'Hmm,' he said. 'Fair point, fair point.'

And with that he went on his way.

Before the match that evening, I'd been to a pub near St Andrews, Birmingham's ground, for a couple of pints. As soon as I had a drink in my hand, a gentle roar went up around me. Several voices piped up with words to the effect of, 'He's off the wagon, look at him.' Or, 'I thought you'd stopped drinking, you lying bastard.' And so on.

In the programme I never said I'd be stopping drinking, but that's what many people seemed to take from it regardless. Because that's how it is with our attitude to alcohol: if you confess to some kind of dependency issue, then you must be an out-and-out drunk, in which case moderation is impossible and complete abstinence the only way forward. I didn't advance this view at the time, obviously; I just said something like, 'Come on, needs must, big game tonight.'

And this seemed to ease their concerns.

None of this bothers me at all, by the way; it's easily dealt with. Rather harder to negotiate are the many people who've sidled up to me in streets or supermarket aisles, on petrol station forecourts or buses, and in pubs or restaurants or doctors' surgeries, or wherever. They gently hold me by the shoulder or hand, look me in the eye, and whisper, 'Good luck with your struggle.' Their faces are a study in kindly concern. I never know what to say to them. I've tried stammering about how I'm just cutting down, but this only elicits pity at my naivety. So I just mumble my thanks and move on.

🍷🥃🍺

I like it best when people say to me that, until they saw the documentary, it had never occurred to them that they might have a problem. And often I'll be told the programme managed to reach a husband, wife or parent in a way that no amount of hectoring down the years has managed to achieve.

I've had people share with me stories of their intake in great detail. How they started drinking and why; when it became a problem; how they stopped; why they started again; how they cut down, and so on. Drinking habits fascinate me. I've met people who drink all day every day and refuse to accept there might be risks associated with this; I met a woman who told me with real feeling how much she looked forward to her only drink of the year, a glass of champagne on her birthday. The drinking club is a broad church indeed.

I bought my sister-in-law a gin-drinkers' advent calendar. She hardly drinks but is partial to the occasional drop of gin. In this calendar was a tiny bottle of gin for each day of advent, which she started working her way through on December 1. She kept telling me it was the best present ever. I was concerned I might have set her on a road to ruin. I needn't have worried; it was midsummer before she got to the bottom of the last miniature bottle, the one marked for Christmas Day.

At the other end of the scale, the day after we'd filmed my dramatic liver scan, I was in a taxi with the TV crew. I could see the driver was listening with vague interest to our conversation, so I asked him how much he drank.

'Twenty-four pints a week,' he said.

'That's a very precise number,' I pointed out.

'Well,' he explained. 'I don't drink during the week because of this job. Then at the weekend I go to the pub. I have twelve pints on Saturday and twelve pints on Sunday. And that suits me,' he concluded firmly, as if daring us to call the wisdom of his boozing regime into question. None of us did.

We were on our way to an interview with an eminent doctor by the name of David Nutt. David's a psychiatrist and professor of neuropsychopharmacology. I'd first met him ten years earlier when he appeared on a show I was presenting. He'd recently run into some controversy in his role as chairman of the government's Advisory Council on the Misuse of Drugs for, essentially, suggesting that some illegal drugs, such as cannabis and even ecstasy, weren't quite as dangerous as many experts claimed.

Trying to be a clever dick in the interview, I told him I'd never taken recreational drugs and wondered which one he'd recommend starting on. 'What's a good entry-level drug for beginners?' I asked. He wasn't going to fall for that one in a hurry and didn't give me an answer, so we moved on.

After the show we gathered in the bar at the studio where I thanked the professor for coming on. 'I thought you said you didn't take drugs?' he demanded.

'Er, I don't.'

'What's this then?' he said, nodding at the glass of red wine in my hand.

Point taken.

Now I was sitting in his office with him, as he frowned at the numbers on the report from my liver scan.

'Hmm,' he said. 'I think you'll have to cut down a bit.'

Again, point taken.

Without much noticing or caring about the irony of it, we agreed to meet for a drink and talk it through.

We got together a week later in a wine bar, and certainly drank slightly more than government guidelines advise. We also, as I remember, ate dangerous quantities of fine cheese. David, like many specialists in this field, is nobody's idea of an evangelical killjoy. Far from it, which is why I tend to trust what he, and others like him, tell me.

I've spoken to a great many doctors and scientists in some depth. Feeling something of a fraud, with only a mediocre degree in English Literature to my name, I've addressed conferences of hepatologists and toured hospital wards, rather fancying myself in the white coats they give me to wear. The majority of medics are absolutely clear that government guidelines have got it about right: that if you drink more than 14 units of alcohol a week, you risk harming your health. If it's a little bit more, or even twice as much, the increased risk is still pretty minimal; if it's a lot more – beyond around 35 units a week – then things can start getting serious for you.

I've met a few doctors who aren't quite so sure about that, and a great many more doctors who don't disagree with the 14 units a week advice, but don't comply with it either. During a long day at Edgbaston Cricket Ground watching England get thrashed by Australia, one doctor I was, er, drinking with, told me that as long as you keep it below 50 units a week, 'You should be fine.'

I've also read a lot of academic research on the physical and psychological effects of alcohol; the relative merits of different countries' approach to legislation; and the effectiveness of different treatments. Many of these papers, I'll admit, are written in a language I struggle to understand, but I've known who to ask for translations. Just thank me for reading them, so you don't have to.

Units, and counting the bloody things

If there's one single reason I've managed to cut down on my drinking, it is because I know how much I'm drinking. I've committed to counting, and keeping a record of, what I've drunk. This is key. It is boring, it is annoying, and it demands a certain dogged commitment to self-flagellation. But if you want to drink less, you must force yourself to do it. You can't calculate how much fuel your car is using if you don't measure how much you're putting into it. You need this data. You need to know how much you are drinking. You have to know your units.

It's amazing how shaky people are about how many units of alcohol there are in whatever they like drinking. Some of the most academic people I know – heads of think tanks, eminent journalists, teachers, chief executives and so on – profess to find the whole concept quite beyond them. 'Remind me,' they plead. 'What is a unit again?' They ask this in a tone which suggests that, try as they might, they just can't quite grasp it. It's the tone of voice I use when I wail that I can't get my head around the American electoral system, or changes to football's offside rule. A doctor I know, who likes a drink himself, told me that the problem with counting units is that they don't allow for different strengths of beer or wine. What? C'mon doc, you know this. The stronger the drink is, the more units there are in it. And there are plenty of apps to help you with the simple calculations necessary.

I put all this confusion down to two things. Firstly, there's the deliberate myopia; drinkers seem to work quite hard to remain as confused as possible. It's easier like this. And the outcome is that many drinkers' heads are buried so deeply in the sand it's a wonder they can get a glass to their lips. Secondly, the alcohol industry doesn't cry into its beer about all this uncertainty. It rather suits them, so they don't do a great deal to help.

To be fair, it can all get a bit complicated if you get too hung up about precision, but the basics are straightforward enough:

- A unit of alcohol is 10ml or 8g of pure alcohol, which is how much you get in a shot of spirits or a very small glass of wine.

- A pint of beer tends to be a bit more than two units.

- If all you drink is whisky, vodka or gin, it's pretty simple. A standard 25ml measure of spirits is one unit.

So, if you drop a single shot of vodka or gin or whisky you have drunk one unit. If you drink a double measure you have drunk, yes, that's right, two units. Well done.

With beer it's less simple as it depends on the strength of the beer. A pint of strongish beer with an ABV (don't worry about what that stands for) of 5.2 per cent is 3 units. A pint of rather weak beer with an ABV of 3.5 per cent is 2 units.

With wine, admittedly, it's trickier still as there's neither standard measures nor glass sizes. A single unit's worth of average strength wine (around 12 per cent) is 85ml. That's such a small serving you could pour it into an espresso cup without any overflow into the saucer. If you were served a measure that small in a pub, you'd probably refuse to pay for it. You're more likely to get 125ml as a standard measure – 1.5 units. If you imagine a half-pint beer glass, that much wine would almost half fill it. A medium measure will most likely be around 175ml, containing 2 units of alcohol; that much would be just short of two-thirds of a half-pint glass. And a large glass of wine may be as much as 250ml, which is more than a third of a bottle, and 3 units worth. Again, the units will depend on the strength of the wine.

At which point, I'm sure you're thinking that I've rather undermined my own claim that it's not very complicated to work out. So, allow me to simplify it all for you; let's do a bit of judicious rounding up or down. It won't hurt; not being accurate to the decimal point is surely better than not counting your units at all. Let's not allow the perfect to be the enemy of the good here.

It's amazing how many people I speak to gave up counting their units because they felt they couldn't do it accurately enough. So, to be clear, they've gone from having never counted their units to being such sticklers for absolute accuracy that they can't bear to continue. If I didn't know better, I'd think it was just another excuse to stick their heads back in the sand.

A rough figure is almost as good as a totally accurate one, and certainly a hundred times better than no figure at all. So, allow me to suggest some shortcuts, starting with beer.

The strongest comes in at around 5.2 per cent, and the weakest at 3.5 per cent. The mid-point is 4.35 per cent. I hereby suggest, without consulting any medic, academic or public health specialist, to count anything below that 4.35 per cent as 2 units a pint, and anything above it as 3 units a pint. I am therefore giving you permission to count Guinness (4.2 per cent), Fosters (4.0 per cent) and Greene King IPA (3.6 per cent) as 2 units a pint. But I'm afraid you'll have to chalk up pints of Stella (c.5.0 per cent), Peroni (5.2 per cent) and Abbot Ale (5.0 per cent) as 3 points. Once more:

● Weaker beer = 2 units a pint
 Stronger beer = 3 units a pint

The strength of wine also varies, generally somewhere between 11.5 per cent and 14 per cent. There are 9 units in a bottle of 12 per cent wine and 10 units in a bottle of 13.4 per cent wine. So, if you can be bothered to check the strength, call it 9 units for a weak wine or 10 for a stronger one. Or just split the difference:

● A bottle of wine = 9.5 units.

Near enough is good enough.

If there's two of you sharing a bottle of wine, then just count half the units in that bottle. If you've had a bit more than your fair share, add a unit; if you've had a bit less take one off. If you're at a party, or around a dinner table with a few people, it's obviously difficult to be precise so just have a stab at how many glasses you've had and call it 1.5 units a go.

♟ ⛉ ▯

Without the drinks industry's efforts to assist us with our unit counting, it would all be very much easier. To read unit values on bottles and cans, you'll generally need very good eyesight, spectacles or, in some cases, specialist magnifying equipment. But at least, after a lot of lobbying, there's information on there somewhere.

Not so if you go into a pub to buy draught beer, or anything else by the glass, where there is often no information about units at all. There's no reason why there couldn't be information on every beer pump along the lines of: one pint = 2.2 units; half a pint = 1.1 units. (Come to that, why aren't the calories on there? After all, if you buy a bag of crisps for the beer to wash down, the calories in the crisps have to be on the packet.)

Who can blame the drinks industry for keeping these numbers out of sight? If all this information was there on display it would surely lead to them selling a bit less product.

There are many apps available to help you count units. They can over-complicate matters by asking you to input precise measurements of quantity and strength but, if you don't get too bogged down in the devilish detail, they are incredibly useful. My favourite one is *Drink Less* which keeps it as simple as possible. You can use it to keep a tediously accurate record, or an easier, rougher one like mine. Either way, just do it. Force yourself. On the *Drink Less* app a reminder pops up every morning at 11am, which is either most welcome or unwelcome depending on what you have to report from the night before.

🍷 🥃 🍺

Another thing (and this is the kind of important advice most medical professionals won't give you): when you first commit to counting, for a couple of weeks carry on drinking as you have been. That way you'll know where you've been at, and, more importantly, as you start drinking less, you'll be able to see where you've come from. This way the graph of your weekly intake on your app will start high before (hopefully) showing a pleasing downward slope. Whereas if you start counting the week you start moderating, full of good intentions, you'll probably post a nice low number which is then likely to rise a little (or a lot, perhaps) in the ensuing weeks. This will be discouraging; better to have big bad blocks on the bar charts to work down from.

Just so you know, my bar chart is not an entirely pretty sight. The overall picture is good; it starts high with weeks of between 50 and 100 units and eases down to around 25 units a week now. I'd rather it was lower, around the 14 unit mark. But just because I generally struggle to get it down to that level doesn't mean that I should give up the whole idea of moderation. This is really important. Too many drinkers see the 14-unit guidance, feel as if they'll never get their intake down to that level, and decide there's therefore no point bothering to cut down at all. As is often the case with drinking, an all-or-nothing attitude prevails. Madness.

There are certainly patchy areas in my drinking data. Sometimes there's a bit of a spike, and there are several weeks where I seem to have mysteriously stopped counting. This will invariably be because I've slipped into drinking too much and accidentally on purpose stopped keeping a record.

If you argue that this makes something of a mockery of the whole process, you'd be making a fair point, but when I see that my record-keeping has become shoddy it's the clearest warning signal for me that I need to reassert control. It doesn't mean I've failed; it just means I've slipped up a bit. I don't beat myself up too much; I merely pat myself on the back for seeing the signs and resolve to tidy things up. My point is that I couldn't wrest back control like this if I hadn't been keeping tabs on my intake in the first place.

I offer this lecture on the importance of counting your units having already admitted that I did no such thing in my first thirty-five years of drinking. And it took nothing less than the making of a big TV documentary to force myself to do so. Horrifying as it was, I'm glad I did. It was good to get my head out of the sand.

Why not stop completely?

I once got talking to a Scottish guy in a pub called The Vine in West Bromwich before a football match. He was a West Brom fan who'd moved to the area from Dunfermline thirty-odd years earlier. His accent was so thick it wouldn't have surprised me if he'd come south only that morning. We got talking about drinking, and how much of it was going on around us that lunchtime. 'It's different down here,' he said gravely. 'People do drink, but where I'm from it's a way of life.'

A way of life. Not just a leisure activity or even a job, but a whole way of life! I thought this was hilarious at the time, but I've since come to realise that, for me, drinking has long been nothing less than a way of life.

I know a great therapist, John McKeown, who's helped a lot of people with their alcohol dependence issues. I told him about the many strategies I've used to moderate my drinking. Having listened to me with interest for a while, he asked, in apparent puzzlement or even exasperation, 'Why put yourself through all this trouble? Why bother? What's so great about drinking that you need to keep going with it?'

These are fair questions, and here's how I try to address them.

First and foremost, alcohol is so woven into the fabric of my life, in all sorts of different ways, that it would take a great deal of unpicking. I wish it wasn't so, but there you are.

One Lent, during which I wasn't drinking, a friend of mine got married. I knew there would be lots of nice people at the wedding but, I'm ashamed to say, I wasn't much looking forward to it because, for me, there wouldn't be drink involved. As it turned out, I had a really good time, but it became startlingly clear how reliant I was on alcohol. It wasn't so much the social interactions I struggled with; the laughing and chatting were no problem. It was weirder than that.

Whenever I needed a break from a conversation, I'd say I was off to get a drink, but there are only so many soft drinks you can be bothered with, so I'd wander off in the direction of the bar without getting a drink. And then I'd get into another conversation, which I'd bring to an end by saying I needed to go to the toilet. But because I hadn't drunk my customary quantity of fluid, I didn't need the toilet. No matter, I took my empty bladder to the toilet anyway. I just stood in there for a couple of minutes, having a bit of a break, marvelling at how alcohol had somehow taken charge of the whole rhythm of my being.

Many people I love and trust tell me it's quite impossible for them to drink in moderation. For them it's a straight choice between all or nothing. They can carry on drinking as they are, or give up completely. For some of these friends it's been a life-or-death decision; the drinking was, or is, killing them. For others it's more a case of not being able to see any purpose in drinking moderately, the whole point of their drinking being to get smashed. The one thing moderation can't help you achieve is oblivion. If anyone tells me it's impossible, or merely pointless, for them to drink moderately, and even dangerous to attempt to do so, it's not for me to tell them otherwise.

There is some persuasive evidence that, even if moderation is the ultimate goal, a few months or even years of not drinking at all might be the way to get there. It's also important to say that if you are a very heavy drinker who experiences significant physical withdrawal symptoms when you don't drink – the shakes, hallucinations, seizures or heaven knows what else – then sudden abstinence is plainly dangerous. If that's you, before you attempt moderation or stopping completely or anything else, you should probably put this book down and make an appointment with your doctor.

On this, a woman called Vicky Sharpe, who's worked for many years in the field of alcohol harm in South Wales, shared the criteria she goes by as to who should attempt moderation and who shouldn't. I've kind of retrospectively applied these criteria to myself, as I was three years ago.

She suggests moderation is worth trying if you:

- Have had enough problems with alcohol to be concerned about drinking even though it's not caused any major life disruption.

Yes, this was me.

- Recognise you have problems with drinking, but do not regard yourself as an alcoholic.

Again, yes.

- Don't have a family history of severe alcohol problems.

Yes.

- Have had alcohol-related problems for less than ten years.

Nope, I think it's more like thirty-five years in my case, but there you go.

- Have not been physically addicted to alcohol, that is you can go for a week or two without taking alcohol or tranquilisers and not experience any unpleasant physical symptoms of withdrawal.

Yes, that's me.

Conversely, she suggests that you need to aim for complete abstinence – probably in a carefully managed way – if you are:

- Physically dependent on alcohol, as above.

- Pregnant or soon might be.

- Suffering with drink-related issues like liver disease and so on.

- In the habit of losing control after even a small amount of alcohol.

- Taking medication that clashes with alcohol.

- Abstinent for a year or more.

I'm pleased to say I score zero out of six there.

While I'm painfully aware of the mayhem alcohol can wreak, I still believe that in society as a whole it does less harm than good. As a social lubricant it has a useful, even vital function. It's a way of bringing people together and that's surely a good thing, but only if it's generally used sensibly and, yes, in moderation. Addictive as it can be, the problem lies less in the thing itself than what we do with it. It's like fire or water. Fire can warm you, keep you alive when it's cold, and cook your food to feed you. But it can consume you too; burn you to a crisp. Similarly, we can't live without water, but we can drown in it too. I'd argue that the same thing applies to religion and the internet and lots more besides. These things can all destroy your life or enrich it. Making sure it does the latter rather than the former is the key thing.

If alcohol really is destroying you – and alcohol itself may well impair your judgement on this – then abstinence is the only sensible route for you to go. But it would be hypocrisy for me to advocate that for everyone. Because, as I look back with some fondness on the first half-century of my life, I think of the countless happy times I've had with a drink inside me. Strangers have become friends; friendships have firmed up; great conversations have been had; dances have been danced, and songs sung. All of which, I know, might have happened if drink hadn't been involved, but it wouldn't have been half as easy.

My friend Frank Skinner, who's not touched a drop for thirty years or more, goes further than this. By nearly every measure, giving up alcohol was the best thing he ever did, but he still speaks of a serious downside: 'My social life never recovered from stopping,' he says. He still misses what he calls the 'white heat' of the craic when drink is involved. Ironically, I would have thought this was less true in his case than anyone else's I can think of. But point taken; it's his call. And I've spoken to many ex-drinkers who take a different view – that their social lives are just as good and often better without touching a drop.

My view is that if you give up alcohol completely you might – might – miss out on a lot of things that you know have given you pleasure. The baby that is your social life could go out with the bathwater. If you're a lifelong drinker, as I was/am, you'll probably find that most of your friends drink too. I was staggered to realise how much this applied to me. I have many friends, some of them very close friends. Let's say as many as fifty. I can only think of one of them, Frank, who doesn't drink at all. I always assumed that this friendship group, which was 98 per cent made up of drinkers, merely reflected society, but that's nonsense. All my friendship group reflects is my own image: the image of a drinker. It turns out that all my life, without realising it, I've been sure to surround myself with other drinkers. Nearly all the new friends I've acquired as I've moved through life are drinkers. I must like it this way; I must need the company and the validation they confer on my life choices.

Whether this is a good or bad thing is beside the point; the reality is that this is what my life looks like and this is what I must work with. If drink is part of all your friends' lives, it's a real challenge to stop drinking completely. If I were to stop drinking completely, things would change. I wouldn't be disowned, and I'd still be in touch with my friends and have good times with them, but it would all be different. I suspect it would feel like we were all still playing at the same snooker club, but I'd now have to play with the cue the wrong way around, or even not play at all; just look on from the sidelines.

It's for this reason I was loath to give up drinking completely. Rightly or wrongly, there would be a social price to pay. If I had to stop drinking, for whatever reason, then obviously I would do it, and most of my friends would be right on board with that. But how much better, and easier, to find a way of cutting down instead? I didn't want to throw the baby out with the bathwater.

John McKeown, my therapist friend, told me that when he stopped drinking, he had to effectively de-friend many people, so associated were they with the damaging drinking life he needed to leave behind. I understand that, but I don't feel the same way about the circle of friends surrounding me, or my relationship with alcohol.

In the society I know, alcohol is a big part of life. If you say it shouldn't be like that, I wouldn't disagree with you, but those seeking to change this reality might as well howl at the moon. Nothing's going to change any time soon, so it's greatly to our advantage if we can find a way of making the bloody stuff work for us, rather than, as is too often the case, the other way around.

Getting served

Like many teenagers, I wanted to get out of the house but didn't have many places to go. Local options were limited. I was raised in Hagley, an overgrown village on the edge of Birmingham and the Black Country. Not much went on, especially during the week. When I was about fifteen my dad told me I was at a difficult age. Difficult because, as he put it, 'You're too young to be at home all the time but not old enough to go to the pub.'

How true that felt. I'm not blaming him, but this was the moment that what I already suspected was confirmed: pubs were the pot of gold at the end of my teenage rainbow. They signified the coming of adulthood and all the carefree fun I took to be associated with that. Pubs were the answer to a perennial question: what shall I do? Above all else, pubs were somewhere to go, something to do.

This is an unintended consequence of the minimum drinking age. It was three long years away – a fifth of my life! – before I could drink legally and it felt like an eternity. A desire was set inside me to ripen like an apple. Alcohol assumed a rock-solid significance, even in its absence. Or, indeed, *because* of its absence. Everything in my life would be better when I could go to pubs and drink. I couldn't wait.

Actually, I didn't wait. None of us did. It became the focus of my and my friends' lives to get served in pubs. We thought of precious little else. This phase lasted so long that feelings associated with it were hard-wired for life. I swear that even now, forty years on, when I go into a pub and don't get queried about my age – which is every time – I get a little thrill.

Word would soon spread around school of any pub within walking distance taking a relaxed attitude to the minimum drinking age. A ragtag crew of pubescent barely-shavers would make their way there on Friday nights. I can still feel the nerves of those evenings. It took a good three-quarters of an hour to walk to The Vine in a nearby village called Clent. The walk home took rather longer, because if you'd got served, you'd be pissed. And if you hadn't, you'd shamble home slowly, a study in despondence.

It didn't help that I found it very difficult to lie. The first time I tried to get served in The Vine, the barman was actually starting to pour the lager before he enquired if I was old enough.

'You old enough?'

'Erm, no,' I said.

'Well fuck off then,' he said, mildly enough.

'What did you say that for, you twat?' asked my friends.

I didn't have an answer for them. They all lied and therefore got served. I walked the walk of shame to the door quite briskly before they saw I was welling up.

On another occasion, I was asked my age at a pub on the outskirts of Swansea where I was on holiday.

'Seventeen and a half,' I said.

Puzzled, the barmaid said, 'Well I can't serve you then, can I?'

'No,' I agreed. And back to our chalet I went.

As I was getting nowhere with this honesty policy, I learned to lie. And I took other steps to make my whole act a bit more convincing. Since I didn't look anywhere near old enough, I resolved to at least learn to act as if I were old enough. I took note of how proper grown-ups conducted themselves at the bar and aped them as best I could.

I called one barmaid 'love'. She gave me a very funny look, possibly because I was blushing hotly with the absurdity of it. A few punters in earshot were sniggering. She must have been in her fifties; I was sixteen. I'm blushing now. I've never called anyone 'love' since.

I noted how some adults were quite specific about what they were ordering, along the lines of, 'Pint of mild in a handled glass please, Tom.' So I started working on variations of this in the mirror at home: Pint of Banks's in a straight glass please Bob; Tennents please Ted, and stick a top on it will you. And so on. A friend of mine called Rich came unstuck in a pub called The Hill Tavern. He marched up to the bar and ordered the strongest ale they had. 'Four pints of Jolly Roger please mate,' he said.

The barman said, 'It's Old Roger, son, not Jolly Roger. On your bike.'

Another evening lay in tatters.

It didn't help that puberty seemed to be taking its time in coming. My friend Martyn and I were discussing getting-served tactics one evening, listening to Genesis in his bedroom. 'The proof of the pudding,' he said sagely, 'is in the shaving.' He was right, and neither of us had much to shout about in that department. It was our understanding that the more you shaved, the quicker your facial hair grew. So I bought a disposable razor, had a squirt of some of my dad's shaving foam, and set about my bum fluff with careful purpose. A fortnight later, to my delight, it needed shaving again.

Another tactic was to acquire older friends. I started hanging around with people who had proper stubble as well as birth dates more than eighteen years previous. Being with them made getting served easier, although I often noticed barmen eyeing me suspiciously. One time I heard a friend being asked, with a nod in my direction, if I was old enough. Quiet words were spoken along the lines of, 'He's with us, don't worry.' Now that's what I call friendship.

One of this gang was a neighbour who I'll call Gary. I had no words to express my gratitude to him for taking me under his drinking wing. I idolised him. We had a couple of drinks in a pub called The Cross Keys one evening. As we walked away, he tapped me on the shoulder and offered me some fatherly advice: 'When you've been sitting in a pub like that, especially when you're underage, it's always a good idea to acknowledge the publican as you leave; you just ignored him then.'

I was mortified. To this day, I never leave a pub without trying to catch the eye of someone behind the bar. These things are important.

🍷 🥃 🍺

A (literally) intoxicating taste of the future came my way in 1983. During the long summer after our O levels, a couple of mates and I went to what was then Yugoslavia. My mum is Croatian, and our family had an old stone house on an island in the Adriatic. This trip held two main attractions for us. There were the girls, and there was the alcohol. We enjoyed more success with one than the other.

If there were any rules about underage drinking in the Federal Socialist Republic of Yugoslavia at that time, nobody applied them. When you asked for a beer, you got one. Under the benevolently severe gaze of President Tito, whose portrait hung in every establishment, we'd glug huge glasses of strong lager quite unable to believe our luck. It was also ludicrously cheap. Even better value were the shots of plum brandy old fellas sold from the back of boats in the harbour. Night after night we got very drunk indeed. It was fabulous.

Nearly forty years on, the three of us are still friends. Rich went on to drink quite dangerous amounts until sorting himself out in his twenties. He still enjoys a drink but seems to have drunk progressively less the older he's got. He now lives in Malaysia where he's got a good job as a project manager. I recently saw him when I had a night in Singapore on my way back from Australia. I actually hadn't drunk for a week and felt good for it, but there was no way on God's green earth either of us could have countenanced meeting up without sharing a couple of beers. This we duly did, and it was a great evening; moderate drinking at its best.

Our third musketeer, Jim, lives in Brighton. He's done very well for himself too, and he too still enjoys a drink. When I last went to see him, he got two bottles of beer out of his fridge and, unbidden, handed one to me. I hadn't planned to drink, and he certainly wouldn't have forced me, but there was no way I could refuse; it would have been like refusing a handshake.

Back on the Adriatic in 1983, while we enjoyed spectacular success in our mission to get pissed out of our heads every night, we did rather less well at wooing girls. I'm afraid we just stared at them, in slack-jawed appreciation of their radiant beauty; no amount of Dutch courage was enough to embolden us to engage any of them in conversation. Actually, I tell a lie. One night, overwhelmed with admiration for a German girl, I did make a move. I knew she was German, not because she told me, but because I had done O level German and had been eavesdropping for several hours. I resolved to break our trio's conversational duck.

'But what shall I say?'

'Offer her a fag,' suggested one of my mates. They felt like my cornermen in a boxing match sending me out onto the canvas. I nodded determinedly and edged my way towards her.

'Möchtest du eine Zigarette?' I ventured, with a confidence only possible if you've downed three shots of plum brandy and two large beers.

She glanced at me without interest, took a cigarette, and carried on chatting to her mate. I never even got a 'danke' out of her, which was a real shame as I was ready with my 'bitte'. I sauntered back to my friends, with a swagger suggesting this encounter represented something of a triumph.

'Well done, Ade,' they said, clapping me on the back. I was still shaking with nerves as we repaired back to the dockside hooch-seller.

We never saw the German girl again.

Furthermore, possibly even at that moment, whoever was marking my O level German paper decided to fail me. This news was conveyed to me by my parents over the phone, the day before we returned home. While I was disappointed, weighing rather more heavily on my mind was the prospect of going back to the stress of age-restricted drinking.

🍷🥃🍺

Back home, when the search for persuadable publicans became too exhausting, there was an alternative route to intoxication which also happened to be cost-effective: home-brewing. It's always seemed most odd to me that while on a Friday evening I could be booted out of a pub for trying to drink underage, the following morning I could emerge from Boots in Stourbridge carrying a home-brewing kit with which to make enough beer to destroy most of the sixth form.

I think our parents might have convinced themselves that home-brewing was allowable as an educational exercise. I made a big show of taking pride in my work, carefully sterilising bottles, reading my hydrometer and knowledgeably sniffing the contents of the large bucket in the airing cupboard. Also, I daresay most adults were aware that the stuff we made tasted so unpleasant it would be a challenge to get enough of it down to achieve any state of intoxication. I can feel that unmistakeable yeast aftertaste gurgling up in the back of my throat even as I write.

Apart from the ghastly taste of the stuff, there was no getting away from the fact that home-brew lacked the illicit pleasure of pub drinking. Where was the joy in doing something that nobody seemed to mind you doing? That said, parental approval was soon withdrawn after a very unpleasant incident concerning some strawberry wine, an ambulance and an overnight stay in hospital for one of my friends.

The home-brewing era had been short and glorious, but it was time for it to end.

Happily, by then our bum fluff was turning bristly and our hit rate for getting served in pubs was moving up past the 50 per cent mark. Even better, off-licences rarely turned us down. The question was now less about whether you could get hold of alcohol, than how much of it you could drink. After all, there was drinking, and there was drinking. It was considered a special achievement, marking you out as a real man, if you could get four cans of Carlsberg Special Brew down. The rules were strict: merely getting it down wasn't enough; you had to get it down and keep it down. Heaving it back up rendered all your efforts null and void. Good try son, but no cigar.

However we did it, whoever we did it with, wherever we did it, drinking was the only thing I wanted my social life to be about. An evening out in which drink didn't feature probably wouldn't happen in the first place: no booze, no point going out.

My friends felt the same way, but many of them had by then started having sex, so their focus shifted a little. I couldn't find anyone interested in having sex with me, so my main interest remained drinking.

This hobby, this passion, this way of life, unhindered by the distraction of anything approximating a sex life, I carried on past my GCSEs and on to my A levels. One of the best things about the lower-sixth year was that we were lumped in with the upper sixth. Among their number were boys who, on reaching the age of eighteen, could get served in pubs.

A school trip to London to see *Hamlet* one weekend was rich with promise as the upper-sixth English students were on the bus too. In the afternoon, ahead of the theatre in the evening, a couple of older lads and I went looking for a pub. For some reason we ended up in the City of London which, with it being a weekend, was very quiet. Accordingly, the pubs were either empty or closed, but we found one called the Viaduct Tavern. (One of the lads I was with, incidentally, is now a barrister in chambers just around the corner.) The three of us drank all afternoon. I felt extremely happy; nothing less than totally fulfilled. This was living. The production of *Hamlet* that evening was at the Shaw Theatre on the Euston Road. I spent nearly all of it in an ecstasy of discomfort, desperate for the toilet.

🍷 🥃 🍺

Most summers I'd be lumbered with a teenager or two from Croatia. My mum had friends, or friends of friends, from Zagreb who had sons around my age who were invited to come and stay with us. I wouldn't have been totally against this if any of them had shown any interest in alcohol. They didn't, something which I found bewildering; I just couldn't get my head around it. I may have wondered if it said more about me than

67

them but doubtless decided otherwise; I concluded there was either something wrong with them or the society they'd grown up in. Or both. It was an idiotic thing to think but, to this day, I catch myself harbouring similar thoughts. I recently asked a friend of mine – who likes a drink herself – how her teenage daughter was getting on. Was she out boozing much?

'No, she doesn't drink,' my friend said.

My first thought, even after everything I now know about drinking, was that there must be something wrong with the poor girl. To be clear, there wasn't.

Going back thirty years, there was nothing wrong with Dražen either. He was one of the many teetotalling teenage guests I struggled to get to grips with. However different their interests were to mine, I could have found a way of getting on with them if they'd shared my passion for alcohol. Dražen was into sport, politics and, to me, unsettling holistic stuff like meditation. I could happily have engaged with him about these or any other passions he might have had, but, without drinking together, it was so much harder. Alcohol was already the portal through which I needed to climb to get into properly empathetic conversations.

As it was, with no drink to bond me with my guests, all they tended to do was to get in the way. Poor Dražen was dragged around on my search for underage drinking opportunities. In his favour was the fact that, unlike me, he looked old enough to get served. I took him to the pub I had taken to describing as my local. I sauntered towards the bar with all the casual confidence I could muster. As I did so, I asked him what he wanted to drink. He shrugged and said, 'some juice'. I was so tense about getting served that it even annoyed me that he said 'some' when he meant 'some kind of'. I really wasn't a very nice young man, at times. My concern was that ordering juice for this lanky Croatian teenager would arouse suspicion. Happily, I still managed to get myself a lager along with his orange juice. We sat there drinking our different drinks. It really was most unsatisfactory.

A few days later, Dražen's non-alcoholic tour of West Midlands pubs took him to a charming country inn, The Swan in Chaddesley Corbett. Somehow, a pint of Batham's bitter ended up in Dražen's hand, and before long he was a bit tiddly. As this group of friends were a bit older, and we were sat in the garden out of sight, getting hold of beer wasn't going to be a problem. What with that, and my guest actually drinking beer, I started to feel really very happy with things. At one stage we started laughing that Dražen was drunk. Grinning a bit inanely he stood up, raised one leg, placed his opposite elbow on the knee and supported his chin with his fist.

'What the fook you doing, mate?' someone asked.

'It is how we show we are not drunk in my country,' he explained. 'Look, I do not fall!'

And we all laughed.

I suppose this tale should end shockingly, with Dražen puking everywhere and never drinking again, or perhaps with him going on to have an illustrious drinking career. Neither is true. What is really shocking though is this: as soon as he had a drink in his hand, I had a real sense of achievement. I felt it was a proper evening, during which we had bonded and become friends. More importantly, I found I really liked him. But on our next visit to a pub, when I asked what he wanted to drink, he shrugged and said 'some juice'. I was dismayed, not to say annoyed. 'Oh come on,' I wanted to say. 'We've been through this; I thought we'd made progress.' I decided we'd never be proper friends after all.

Dražen is the son of an old friend of my mum's. He's a nice guy, intelligent and funny, and his interests aren't (and never were) a million miles from mine. If he'd been any kind of drinker we would quite definitely have been firm friends.

Every time I went to Zagreb I'd have called him up and bonded afresh over a few beers. But because he didn't drink, I tended not to look him up and gradually acquired other friends in Zagreb who I really treasure. They too are nice, intelligent, interesting people and, entirely coincidentally I'm sure, they all like a drink.

The last time I saw Dražen was, randomly, in some kind of temple when I was working in Delhi for a few days. He was teaching yoga there and was really happy, and plainly still didn't need alcohol to be so.

The Swan in Chaddesley Corbett featured heavily in my A-level year. Most lunchtimes in the upper sixth I'd drive down there with a mate or two. I'd have a pint of Batham's and a chicken and mushroom pie. It was part of my routine. On my eighteenth birthday the barmaid brought out a chicken and mushroom pie with a candle stuck in it. I could now drink legally, not that by then it made much difference.

I was in the school production of the musical *Cabaret*. I played one of the main characters, the American, Cliff Bradshaw. Mr Fenwick, a chemistry teacher, played the MC. After rehearsals I'd give him a lift (I'd just passed my driving test) to Stourbridge Junction station and, thrillingly, we'd go for a pint at a pub next to it called The Labour In Vain. We talked about all manner of stuff. These quick pints with an intelligent adult felt like nothing less than the first concrete foundations for adulthood.

It was also the first time that I had ever heard a teacher swear. Mr Fenwick was recalling how scared he'd felt during the Cuban missile crisis. 'I was thinking, "Fucking hell there's going to be a nuclear war,' he told me, "and we're all going to die".'

Drinking beer, talking about adult stuff and real feelings with a proper bloke. It felt wonderful. But, again, the beer was what seemed to make it happen.

My favourite teacher was Mr Ralph, who taught English. He was a wonderful, inspiring man and, in ways he probably didn't realise, a great life coach. One time after a concert at school I gave him a lift home. I was pissed off with something disparaging a parent had said to me about my double bass playing as we were leaving. 'Well, you gave them all a good laugh anyway,' were her exact words. I shared this with Mr Ralph, who was very supportive. In fact, sweetly, he said he had more to say than we had time for on this short journey and he suggested popping for a drink somewhere.

'It's quarter to eleven,' I said, puzzled.

'Oh, is that too late?'

'Yes, course, they close at half ten in the week.'

'Oh,' he said.

It never occurred to me that anyone could not know that was the case; it was the law of the land at the time and, as far as I was concerned, as commonly known as the fact that the sun rose in the east. But Mr Ralph, who seemed to me to know an awful lot about everything, obviously wasn't a drinker. I might have taken this as an indication that you didn't need to be a drinker to be brilliant. But as it was, I just felt a bit disappointed in him.

As a kind of topping-out ritual for our non-drinking teenage years, many eighteenth birthdays were spent doing something called 'The Bathams Eight'. Bathams was and is a fine local ale brewed in Brierley Hill in the middle of the Black Country. At the time there were, famously, only eight pubs selling it. The idea was to get around all eight of them in one evening, taking a pint in each establishment. This took some doing as we were still in the era of pubs not opening until 7pm. Therefore this stern test of logistical planning and drinking capacity could only be attempted on a Friday or Saturday when pubs were open until eleven.

It was widely accepted that to be in with a chance of pulling it off, you had to be in the car park of The Lamp in Dudley at 6.55pm. Upon the doors being unlocked we'd all crowd in and neck our pints with great haste.

'Doing the eight?' the barman would normally enquire, unnecessarily; of course we were.

Heaven knows how minibus drivers were persuaded to work this route. The risks of rattling a load of kids from pub to pub in an old bus were surely obvious. The craic would be phenomenal to start with and get even better as the evening went on, perhaps peaking on the journey between the fifth pub, in Kidderminster, and the sixth, in Kinver. Thereafter, thanks to a queasy combination of bendy country roads and six pints of strong ale, things started to get very quiet indeed.

Arrival at pub number seven, The Plough in Shenstone, generally featured the minibus coming to an abrupt stop, a door being flung open, and a stream of puke emanating from within, closely followed by its issuer. There were fallers at this seventh fence for sure, but a majority would arrive at the eighth and final pub with jaws dead set in determination and a sporting chance of ingesting that last pint, keeping it down, and bathing in the glory of triumph.

This final stop happened to be The Swan, my A-level pub. I still occasionally pay a visit to this delightful place, but always tread gingerly across the car park, grimly aware of just how much evidence lies underfoot of narrowly failed attempts to drink, and hold on to, the Bathams Eight.

Sixth-form drinks scorecard

● POSSIBLE INTERVENTIONS

By now the rot, or perhaps I should call it joy, had set in.
I doubt anyone could have said or done anything to set
me on a different path. It's frightening to consider what it
would have taken to put me off drinking, even at this young
age. It would have to have been something really dramatic:
a serious illness, awful accident or losing my virginity and
falling in love with a teetotaller. Shocking as this is, I'm not
sure I'd have wanted to change anything. It felt great. And
it's not as though I can think of anything I wished I'd been
doing instead, apart from sex, obviously, which wasn't
happening. Perhaps I was drinking as a substitute for sex,
but then I had plenty of mates who drank as much as me
and were having lots of sex too. The lucky bastards.

● CONSUMPTION

I wasn't drinking every day, obviously, although the total
number of days a year I did drink increased year upon year.
No weekends were without alcohol; most would involve
several cans or pints of beer plus some pre-drinking of
vodka or some such. I reckon that over a weekend I'd be in
for about eight pints of beer plus five measures of some
spirit or other and the odd glass of wine at home. Let's say
20-25 units a week.

● BORING BITS

They were beginning to creep in. There might be more
boring times than I remember, because boring times fade
in the memory rather faster than good times. I only felt – or
told myself I felt – bored when I wasn't drinking. Alcohol was,
after all, in my daft young mind, an antidote to boredom.
Apart from anything else, I was breaking the law for most
of this time, so that always gave it a certain frisson. Also, it

still felt new, and made me think that lots of exciting things were possible, which is not something I tended to think when not drinking.

Every Friday night, the Stone Manor, a local country house hotel near Kidderminster, would have a disco. With great excitement, booze would be procured to drink before we got there, and the older-looking among us were deployed to get drinks in once we were inside. Looking around at the girls who might fancy me, and cool boys who'd want to hang out with me, the possibilities seemed endless. The more I drank, the more imminent it felt that my hopes would come to fruition. This thrilling feeling would last until around two-thirds of the way through the evening. At that point it started to become apparent that few, if any, of my fantasies were coming true. It was then that boredom and unhappiness would kick in.

The Stone Manor, sweetly, laid on free curries of unspecified meat towards the end of the night. With drink having failed to deliver on its promise to bring joy, or even merely alleviate boredom, I instead sought solace in these food offerings. I'd eat myself to a standstill before sloping off home.

In the morning I'd pick gristle from between my teeth and assess my hangover. I'd feel a bit idiotic but, unaccountably, by lunchtime, the potential for joy when I next drank would already be crowding into my head. This is the puzzling thing. The boredom – what I'd been drinking to avoid in the first place – had somehow been forgotten. I suppose that's the problem with boredom: it's too easily forgotten. Or maybe this is a key, dangerous component of the drug that is alcohol: it leaves you unable to recall boredom.

● PROPORTION OF DRINKS WANTED/NEEDED/ENJOYED

80 per cent.

A drink problem? Me?

The vast majority of drinkers like me believe they are not problem drinkers. Because we don't conform to the stereotype of the 'alcoholic' – drinking in the morning, passing out in the street etc. – we don't think we're addicted to, or dependent on, alcohol. We don't believe we have a drink 'problem'.

What we do have is an answer ready for anyone who accuses us of having a drink problem. This will be in the form of a sentence beginning something like this:

'Me? A drink problem? No! Why, I…'

We finish this sentence in all sorts of imaginative ways. My own ending of choice was:

'Me? A drink problem? No! Why, I… *hardly ever get drunk.*'

I've used countless others too.

Here's a selection. Do help yourself, please.

Me? A drink problem? No! Why, I…

… hardly ever drink during the day.
… usually only drink at the weekend.

... have plenty of days off.

... only drink Saturdays, all day.

... never drink on my own.

... don't drink in the morning.

... do Dry January ever year.

... drink every day, but only a little bit.

... drink every other day.

... only drink when I'm thirsty.

... don't start drinking until it's late.

... stop drinking before it gets too late.

... only drink after work.

... never drink after work.

... don't drink on work nights.

... don't drink during Lent.

... only drink socially.

... only ever drink a little at a time.

... never vomit.

... never pass out.

... always get home.

... never drink spirits.

... only drink wine.

... only drink fine wine.

... never get hangovers.

... never mix drinks.

... know when to stop.

... never miss it when I don't drink.

... am just a binge drinker.

... am just a social drinker.

... only drink because I have to for work.

... only drink at home.

... only drink in pubs.

... never go to the pub.

... don't even like the taste.

… just like the taste.
… could stop any time but I just don't want to.

Use the space below to add any other endings you've heard or used yourself:

Urge surfing

Always on the lookout for new techniques to aid moderation, I was intrigued by something a psychologist mentioned to me called urge surfing.

I looked it up and read that:

Urge surfing is a mindfulness technique used to get through an urge without acting on destructive impulses. When you notice an urge, rather than fighting against it, imagine you are on a surfboard riding with it. Notice the shifting sensations, how they rise and fall, come and go.

Worth a try.

One hot summer's afternoon when the desire for a cold lager in a pub garden all but overwhelmed me, I got on my mental surfboard to ride the wave of my lager urges. I closed my eyes to visualise the scene, but all I could see on the inside of my eyelids was the front of my surfboard arrowing through a refreshingly cold sea of Stella Artois. I tried some fancy surfing tricks, to try to show my mastery of these waves of desire, but secretly I was hoping to take a tumble and fall right into this sea of cold lager. And in I fell; I couldn't help myself.

When I opened my eyes the thought of a pint of Stella seemed as nothing compared to what I'd just been through, thrashing around in a sea of the stuff. The thirst for that pint had faded away. My urge surfing had worked, albeit not quite in the way it's intended to, but there you go. Worth a try.

What happened when I went to an AA meeting

There were ten of us in the meeting. I asked the facilitator, effectively the chair, if I could say a few words as to what I was doing there.

I said, 'Hello everyone; my name's Adrian.'

'Hello Adrian,' they intoned, as one.

Oh God yes, I thought. I've seen this on films. Wasn't this when I was supposed to say that I'm an alcoholic? Would I get thrown out if I didn't?

'Erm, well, I'm not an alcoholic,' I said. 'At least I don't think I'm an alcoholic.' I was listening to myself talking, rather than talking myself. 'But I do drink an awful lot and couldn't imagine not drinking. I'm not drinking at the moment as it happens, for Lent, and I suppose I'm asking myself the question.'

What question exactly, I did not specify, because I'd never really thought of it like that, but, now that I'd mentioned it, I suppose I was half-asking if I was an alcoholic too.

The attendees beheld me sympathetically, balefully, blankly. Some smiled, others didn't. Nobody objected. The next hour will stay with me forever. I was transfixed. I'm not sure what my expectations or assumptions about the meeting had been, but I'm pretty sure they were confounded. It was all more dramatic than I thought it would be, and yet more mundane too.

This had all come about following a chat in a coffee shop with a producer of a TV panel show on which I was booked to appear. Even though (or most likely because) I wasn't drinking for Lent, drinking was very much on my mind, so we soon got onto the subject. It turned out that she was a long-time attendee of Alcoholics Anonymous. I listened, fascinated, to her story. I remember her saying, 'The main thing was that whenever I drank, I became quite an unpleasant person. I really didn't like myself.' This seemed to me as good a reason as any for knocking your drinking on the head.

When we next met, at the recording of the show, I asked her if I could come along to a meeting. And so it was that I found myself in a dilapidated room in an unloved community centre next to a primary school somewhere in the London suburbs. Around the table were my producer friend, the AA facilitator/chair, a woman in her thirties of South Asian heritage, a man in his sixties with an American accent, and a well-spoken English woman wearing a Barbour. None of the other three people in the room uttered a word. One was a guy in a bandana who stared at the table in front of him and never moved a muscle.

The first person to speak was the woman in her thirties. She made only passing mention of her drinking before embarking on a long, rambling moan about what a terrible place the world was, mainly, in her view, because of bankers. This all seemed a bit off-point and the radio programme host in me was getting impatient. It felt like it all needed moving along a bit. I looked for signs of exasperation on the face of the facilitator, hoping he'd wrap her up, but nothing doing. It doesn't work like that apparently; you talk for more or less as long as you want. Eventually she ran out of steam. No-one said anything.

Next up was the well-spoken woman in the Barbour. She told us that she'd been sober for three months, to murmurs of congratulation. But then she told us how she'd woken up at four o'clock that morning and started thinking about her son, which had led her to go downstairs, open a bottle of wine, and drink it all. She went on to explain the circumstances which had led her to be estranged from her son. The details weren't clear because she started to struggle to get her words out. But the awful essence of it was that he'd been taken away from her because of suggestions she'd abused him in some way.

'I didn't though,' she sobbed. The sound of children from the school playground next door reached us in the room where, by now, the poor woman was howling. 'But I don't know if I did or not because I was drinking so much.' She fell as silent as the rest of us. I realised that my lips had dried up. I wondered if I'd even drawn breath. A tissue was passed to her and we moved on.

The whites of my eyes must have been apparent to the next speaker, the guy with the American accent. He told us that his drinking had never really adversely affected him; he'd been successful in his working life, holding down big jobs which had taken him around the world. He'd been married, as he put it, too many times, but gave the impression this had been nothing to do with his drinking. He described himself as a 'topper-upper' – 'always drinking, never drunk,' he explained. Everything was fine, he said, until a year earlier doctors had taken a look at his liver and told him that if he didn't stop drinking, he would soon die. So, he'd stopped drinking. Before this diagnosis, he'd never considered himself a problem drinker.

This sounded very much like territory I could one day wander into: constant heavy drinking with no obvious side effects until it was almost too late. It was like he was speaking directly to me, which, as it happens, is exactly what he did next.

'Adrian,' he began, his eyes gently boring into my soul. 'You're probably already realising that no two alcoholics are the same: we're all different. All we have in common is that we've drunk too much for too long.'

I nodded and opened my mouth to say something, but nothing came out. If I'd been able to summon words, even only two words, they would have been, 'Point taken'.

After the meeting, as we made our way out, the American approached me, smiling, a study in non-judgemental kindness. 'I've been sober for a year now,' he said. 'And after a year we're supposed to give a copy of the book to someone we think might need it.' And he handed me a blue hardback book with the words 'Alcoholics Anonymous' on the cover. I thanked him, and wanted to talk more, but suddenly we were going our separate ways.

I live several miles from where the meeting was held but, the following morning, as I was driving near my home, I saw the American walking down the road. I pipped my horn and waved but he didn't see me. I looked forward to bumping into him again and having a chat, but I've not seen him since.

I read the book – the basic text of Alcoholics Anonymous, written by its founder in 1939. Though I'm a practising Catholic, and a believer in faith, I couldn't quite get my head round the theological aspect of it. Neither could I buy into the requirement specified at the outset that I should accept I was powerless over alcohol. Of course I had power; of course I had agency. Why, I wasn't drinking this Lent, for a start. And when Lent finished, things would be different. Even if I was kidding myself, I felt it would be worse, dangerous even, to believe that I had lost all control. Apart from anything else, it could have provided an excuse to embark on a bender – don't blame me mate, it's not my fault! I'm not in control!

While there are aspects of AA's philosophy I struggle with, I suspect the meetings do much more good than harm. A friend of mine, a cameraman I worked with, was a problem drinker. After years of chaos in his life he was finally persuaded to go to a meeting. He told me he was terrified at the prospect, a feeling which didn't leave him when he walked into the room, somewhere in the City of London. A well-dressed, executive-looking woman seemed to be in charge. He felt sure she would soon be bollocking him for his terrible behaviour, and was staggered when she began by simply saying what her name was and telling everyone she was an alcoholic.

At that moment, everything changed for him. Because this was the first person he'd come across with similar addiction issues to his own but who was apparently successful with it. This made all the difference to him. He kept going along. It helped. He got put off by the religious stuff, stopped going, and then started going again. He fell off the wagon and reboarded it, but, the last I heard, he was doing OK. Whatever works, or even just works a bit, is no bad thing.

There's something that smartly dressed woman said at the first meeting which stuck in my friend's mind. And once he'd shared it with me, it stuck in my mind too. It was high summer at the time. She talked about how, when it was hot, she'd always struggled to resist the temptation of a cold beer. She described being tormented by the mental image of an ice-cold pint of lager, deliciously decorated with condensation, sitting on a table in a beer garden, just begging to be drunk.

Then she described how she'd forced herself to focus on an alternative image of the pint glass. This one sat on the same table but had contained her fourth or fifth pint, rather than the first. It was half empty, with lipstick smudges around its rim. The condensation had evaporated; the lager was warm. A wasp or two buzzed around it. She found that concentrating on this image instead of the first one was a great help to her. It's a trick I play on myself from time to time. It's worked for me too when I could really do with having a dry summer's evening.

The AA devotee I've met most recently was a middle-aged bloke with a couple of dogs who stopped me in a park in Plymouth. He told me how grateful he was for the work I'd done on drinking. This is obviously nice, but especially when it comes from a recovering alcoholic, a firm abstainer. I always fear their disapproval, worrying that they'll see all my talk of moderation as naïve or even dangerous. Some do; this man didn't. He told me he'd not touched a drop in fifteen years and credited AA for helping him achieve this.

We talked a bit about the merits of AA, specifically how he kind of ignored what he called 'the religious stuff'. We also discussed if he could have cut down instead of stopping completely. On this he said, 'By the end, probably not. Maybe if someone had got to me a bit earlier, who knows?' He concluded our exchange that autumn morning by saying, 'AA is just about throwing the towel in really, isn't it?'

Good metaphor. That's how I see Alcoholics Anonymous and abstinence generally. And to be clear, there's no shame attached to throwing in the towel. When a boxer's trainer physically throws in the towel, it's not done lightly. But when they judge their fighter to be beaten, it has to be done. The safety of the fighter is paramount, be their opponent a boxer or the booze. Whoever or whatever the fight is against, it's obviously for the best if the fighter has trained enough to have acquired the tools and know-how to keep things from getting so desperate. Boxers will do all they can to avoid reaching the stage when the towel needs to be thrown in; drinkers need to think the same way. A key part of this is understanding that there are ways of addressing excessive drinking before that drinker is close to hitting the canvas.

That's certainly the view of Susan Laurie, author of *From Rock Bottom to Sober Forever: How a hopeless alcoholic found complete freedom from her addiction*. I met her when I gave evidence to the House of Lords Commission on Alcohol Harm. Her book is as compelling an account of a descent into what she calls hopeless alcoholism as any I've come across.

One scene sticks out for me. Susan, then in her thirties, was determined to show her husband and son that she had her drinking under control. She decided a good way of doing this would be to cook them a nice meal, even though she was blind drunk at the time. 'This,' she recalls, 'is how my insane alcoholic mind worked.' With devastatingly twisted logic, she decided to demonstrate her soundness of mind and body by cooking a tricky dish. Gratin dauphinoise demands the slicing of potatoes very thinly with the use of a razor-sharp mandoline.

Susan can remember neither cutting off the end of her little finger nor passing out in bed. Her husband arrived home to a kitchen covered in blood. Their son was in his room, upset and angry. Calamities like this were something they, and many of Susan's friends, had witnessed countless times before. Once again it was decided that this would be the last straw; the drinking had to stop. Once again, the drinking didn't stop.

In every other aspect of her life Susan had enjoyed great success. Born in County Durham, she'd been a high achiever at school and after university went on to enjoy a successful career in the pharmaceutical industry. Her dependence on alcohol cost her that career and her first marriage. Neither Alcoholics Anonymous nor hypnotherapy nor counselling sessions nor stints in rehab worked for her.

One of her problems with AA, interestingly, was that listening to other people's stories made matters worse. Tales of their terrible experiences merely led her to conclude that her case was in comparison relatively mild. And this was all the encouragement she needed to get back on the bottle.

By the end, her intake was so wildly out of control that she had resigned herself to an early death. In what amounted to a last throw of the dice she gave hypnotherapy one more try, with a new therapist. She credits him, and a near-death experience in a car crash around that time, with saving her life.

Susan is someone else I was worried would scorn a book about drinking less, but she couldn't be more supportive. She doesn't see anything inevitable or predetermined about her journey to the bottom:

There are so many people who accidentally sort of get sucked down the wrong route. If there was some sort of guidance, you know in a book or whatever, before it gets like that, a lot more people would realise that they are drinking excessively and could end up like I was. If I'd had that kind of guidance, I really don't think I would ever have got as bad as I was.

For me, Lent's abstinence finished a couple of weeks after my brush with Alcoholics Anonymous. After Easter Mass I went for a couple of pints of Guinness with a bloke I met in the church, a cabbie called Mick. It was nice. I felt that my drinking was under control and things were still on course to be different, which they were for about a week. Then, with remarkable speed, I went back to drinking as much as I ever did.

Drink Like Helen B. Merry

Many years ago, I did some amateur drama at a theatre in Birmingham. A leading light of the company was an older woman, a great actor. She looked and sounded like she smoked a lot. Everywhere she went she carried with her a portable ashtray. It had kind of wings of weighted leather, so it could be draped over the arm of a chair. The ashtray was the size of a pocket watch and had a flip-up lid, upon which were engraved the words, 'Smoke Like Helen B. Merry'.

I spent many enjoyable evenings hanging around with this woman, watching her tap ash into her little ashtray. I was a bit in awe of her. I puzzled over those words on the lid. Then one time, doubtless emboldened by drink, I asked her, 'Who is this Helen B. Merry?'

She laughed that hoarse smokers' laugh which is three-quarters mirth and a quarter cough. You don't hear laughs like that so much anymore.

'Idiot,' she wheezed. 'Smoke. Like. Hell. And. Be. Merry.'

'Oh,' I said, mortified. I must have read it a hundred times without noticing.

I've had Helen B. Merry in my head for more than thirty years. I'd never had a use for her until it came to naming this chapter, which is about the health risks associated with drinking. Look, I'm sorry, but if I'd called it 'Health Risks of Drinking', you wouldn't have read it.

I'll keep it brief.

Here's what it boils down to: if you habitually drink more than 14 units of alcohol a week, you're likely to be harming yourself. If you're drinking only slightly more than 14 units, the risk of harm is only slightly elevated. If you're drinking twice as much, the chance of problems developing will obviously be greater. And if you're caning it at a rate of three, four or five times 14 units a week – as I was – then your chances of getting seriously ill grow exponentially. And my understanding of what that means is this: if you double your intake from 30 units a week to 60, you more than double the risk of harm. But, to put a more positive spin on that, if you reduce your weekly intake from 60 units to 30, you are more than halving the risk of harm. Which is good.

There are mountains of scientific studies on all this; some draw slightly different conclusions than others. But having done a fair amount of reading and listening on the subject, I'm pretty confident very few specialists in the field would disagree wildly with my summation.

I should also stress again that I've yet to meet anyone working in this field who doesn't enjoy a drink themselves. When they talk me through the statistics on drinkers' health risks, they usually do so in a tone which says, 'Look, I wish it wasn't so, but I'm afraid it is'. The point is that purveyors of these dark warnings are not, as they're often portrayed in the media, wild-eyed evangelising teetotallers, intent on destroying the alcohol industry. Admittedly, I'm yet to be invited on the Alcohol Harm Specialists' Annual Pub Crawl (there isn't one), but I've had the odd glass with many of them.

A key point that they're always keen to stress is something worrying, and counter-intuitive, about alcohol harm: the majority of those who develop serious problems are not the heaviest drinkers. Most of them are less heavy drinkers. Drinkers like me. Those who drink enormous amounts – pretty much all day every day – are obviously more likely, individually, to get ill. But numerically they're not the biggest part of the problem. It's the quarter of drinkers getting through between 14 and 50 units a week who are becoming ill in the biggest numbers. Because there are more of us.

So, if you are like I was – the heavy drinker who walks past the guy lying in the shop doorway and thinks you'll never get as ill as him – be aware that there are more drinkers like you than there are like him on liver wards.

The problem drinkers like me often have (being apparently OK health-wise despite what we're putting away) is that our early warning systems tend not to be functioning properly. I played golf at a charity day with a former Tory MP called Anthony Coombes. Our conversation turned to alcohol. He told me he wasn't much of a drinker. 'I do drink a bit,' he said. 'But not that much because, fortunately, I'm blessed with hangovers.'

Blessed. This was nicely put. He didn't drink much, simply because if he did, he felt bloody awful in the morning. I wish I was more like him. My problem was that I rarely got hangovers, or indeed any other obvious adverse reaction to large amounts of alcohol. So in the absence of any pressing health issues, I'd carry on drinking vast amounts. Even one colossal hangover might have encouraged me to put on the brakes, as would a drunken fall and a shaming visit to a casualty ward. Something, anything, might have been helpful. But everything was apparently fine until I had that liver scan for that TV programme.

Drinkers like me often end up in trouble precisely because we don't display many of the obvious side effects of heavy drinking, such as terrible hangovers, florid complexions, huge beer bellies and so on. We can fly under our own radar, which is a risky way to proceed.

On the other hand, there had been enough warning signs if I'd only chosen to take them on board. For years, I've been taking daily medication prescribed for those three middle-age maladies: anxiety/depression, hypertension and reflux. I'd never really associated my drinking with any of them. This was silly because alcohol is the biggest known cause of hypertension; as a depressant it obviously has negative psychological impacts; and it's known to be detrimental to gastric health.

That I chose not to make these links is down to me, but it's not as if any of the specialists I consulted had much to say on the subject either. While all the gastroenterologists, cardiologists, psychologists and psychiatrists who treated me did ask about my alcohol consumption, none of them seemed to set much store by it. If they thought alcohol might be at the root of my problem – or, at least, one of the causes – in their particular specialism, they didn't share that with me. I took this to mean they were fairly relaxed about it, seeing excess drinking as an unfortunate fact of life which couldn't be avoided anyway, so best not to worry about it.

Or maybe that's just what I wanted to think they thought.

Mea culpa, probably. When it came to my drinking, if my head wasn't buried in a pint, it was, as ever, generally buried in the sand.

His name is Bryn and he is a moderator

It's hard to find people who've successfully moderated their alcohol intake. This might be because very few of us actually manage to do so. It might also be because it's not generally considered something to shout about. As I've said, while you often hear of people quite rightly celebrating anniversaries of their sobriety, you never hear of anybody having a moderation celebration party.

Unlike abstinence which is, if nothing else, clear, the whole business of moderation is shrouded in greyness. Like abstinence, it has a beginning – or several false starts – but, unlike abstinence, it has no clearly defined end. All of which, to my mind, makes it at least as great an achievement as stopping completely.

Just as there's no precise measure of success, there is no single route to success. From my research, I suggest that different methods, ideas, thoughts and tricks work, or don't work, for different people at different times. As everyone drinks for different reasons at different times in different ways, it's hardly surprising that successful moderators have all managed to pull it off in all sorts of different ways.

Of all the successful moderators I've spoken to, I've chosen four for this book – each of whom have had different relationships with alcohol and therefore different routes to drinking less of it. Here's the first of their stories.

🍷 🥃 🍺

Bryn Jones, in his seventies, is an academic based in Bath. He used to drink around 50 units a week but is now down to single figures and has been for a long time. As we support the same football team, I'd been on nodding terms with Bryn for twenty-odd years.

Then he sent me a rather brilliant email.

I too have been down the road on which you now find yourself, although I embarked on it a bit earlier in the life cycle. Somehow, without outside intervention, I blundered into a modus vivendi with alcohol that I've now managed to sustain for quite a few years.

I'm also lucky that my occasional dabbling in social psychology, as an academic, has given me helpful ideas to make sense of it all. If I were to give a talk on reducing involvement in heavy social drinking it would go something like this.

To climb out of the enjoyable mire of constant drinking one needs three things:

an intellectual rationale for giving up the present way of life;

an overall strategy that demotes drinking from its undeserved pedestal in your life;

a set of techniques for staying on drier land when the torrents of booze can, almost literally, drown you.

'Undeserved pedestal.' I like that very much; well said, sir. Immediately I have an image of myself genuflecting before a pedestal. Atop this pedestal sits a pint of Guinness or cold lager and a glass of wine. Because, absurdly, my attitude to these things has amounted to nothing less than veneration. I've thought they'd make me happy, console me, make a good night great and a bad night tolerable. I've believed they enhance my life. And even if they do, a bit, in some ways, they still don't deserve to be up there on that pedestal.

As you've pointed out, we don't seem to have an accepted code for regulating our drinking anymore. It's available almost everywhere and anywhere at any time. Popular culture is much more permissive of unrestricted drinking than it was 100 years ago, or even when you and I were growing up. With tacit help from the media (typical interviewer question to successful match winners: 'Suppose you'll really be out for a few drinks celebrating this win tonight?'), it's become an accepted way of life; provided, as you pointed out, the drinker doesn't get violent, abusive or vomit over bystanders.

I think it's helpful if we develop coherent social or ethical arguments for not accepting this way of life. For example, it might help you quit smoking if you consider the vast profits made by Big Tobacco. It's similar with alcohol: every time we have a booze-up, we are legitimising the consumption they actively promote via their huge economic power and considerable political influence. We set examples for everyone else, and unwittingly reinforce the kind of lifestyle which lines Big Alcohol's coffers.

I channel this kind of anger a lot. As I've already banged on about, I've only got to look at a beer pump and see the absence of information on there to get riled up. Why doesn't it say how many units there are in a pint of the stuff? Or, even more importantly, the calories? It annoys me no end, and this annoyance is a great help when I'm deciding whether, or how much of the stuff, to drink.

In the spirit of summoning up my righteous indignation, Bryn even suggests channelling religion:

I was brought up as a Methodist, so the demon drink was always an uneasy companion. However, living with an ex-Catholic, I know that you Catholics are much less condemnatory and more forgiving of over-indulgence, but I'm sure there must be some critical doctrine against boozing?

Hmm, not sure about that, unfortunately.

What would Jesus do? Well probably more likely to transform wine into water than the other way around, if He came back today.

That's a can of theological worms I don't want to open. Let's not go there.

All I'm trying to say is that some sort of intellectual perspective that is critical of frequent drinking does help, or at least helped me and motivated me to be less enthusiastic about my drinking.

What I did some years ago was to say to myself: daily drinking is counterproductive, so on what days of the week could I most easily abstain? You might be surprised to read that the first target was match days, specifically the ritual of the pre-match rounds. So that meant turning up a bit later, or going straight to the ground instead of the pub. And I was pleasantly surprised at how enjoyable it was to observe exactly what was happening on the pitch, instead of viewing it through an alcoholic fog. I saw more. I learned more. I remembered more. Nowadays I sometimes meet the lads at the pub before a game, but nobody is sniffy that I'm one of the few drinkers on tomato juice or fizzy water.

Weekdays. I began finding other things to do until about 9 or 10 pm. That left just enough time for a single nightcap, which I enjoyed all the more as my deserved treat.

This works especially well for me, because whenever I tell myself I'm saving myself for a late drink, by the time I get there I often don't bother. This was how I gave up smoking, many years ago. I'd not have a cigarette all day on the promise to myself of having one smoke last thing, just before bed. I really looked forward to that cigarette all day, even though I knew that, when the time came, I'd ask myself if I really needed it and, so close to bedtime, would decide I didn't. I'd then promise myself I'd have one the next day last thing before bed. And so on.

With drink, the challenge for me is different. It's the early evenings I struggle with, when I can think of nothing else in the world I want more than a quick pint. If I can get past that hump, I'm generally fine. Anyway, back to Bryn.

Gradually it became about avoiding any drink during the working week which, happily, resulted in my aptitude and appetite for work increasing dramatically. Weekends were more problematic. By then my drinking was pretty much restricted to Friday and Saturday nights, but these often resembled a drinking competition or some binge drinkers' carnival.

Yes, I've attended that carnival on several occasions. If it was a real carnival, I could see myself on a float.

Now I'm down to two to three pints on these nights, and my drinking is confined to the pub. Only occasionally would bottles of wine be opened at home. I've stuck to this regime for twenty years now, apart from special occasions like Christmas and so on. But even then I drink less than I used to, because as you reduce the intake you need less to get the same effect.

Less. Is. More. If only we drinkers could get that in our stupid heads and keep it there.

So that's the ethical framework and the strategy. What about the nitty gritty of the occasion? There are some techniques I've found useful. I ration pub drinking to a couple of hours in the evening. It's good to set a finishing time and keep to it. My own practice is to not go to the pub till about 9pm. Tiredness and the morning regime then dictate I have to leave before midnight. Also, I tend to have my biggest meal of the day before I go out. That way the stomach is still full at the pub and the gut's space for large volumes of fluid is reduced. A full stomach also tends to soak up some of the alcohol. Then there's the actual process of consumption. Here are my tips:

Cut out high alcohol beers. There's lots of excellent bitters and IPAs at less than 4 per cent volume. Four pints of 3.6 per cent beer contain fewer units of alcohol than three pints of 5.0 per cent beer.

I tend to go one step further than this and ask for a pint which is half beer and half soda water. This, obviously, gives you half the units of whatever beer you make it with. So, two pints of 5 per cent lager – and taste-wise it's best to make it with a strong beer – comes in at less than three units rather than nearly six. To my mind, it barely tastes any different to the real thing. And, importantly, you have a pint to hold.

The only problems I've had with this approach are all the fault of the licensed trade. It's often difficult to make it understood what you are ordering, as this concoction has no name I know of. I've settled upon saying it's 'like shandy, but made with soda instead of lemonade.' That seems to work. The other challenge is getting over your annoyance that you'll most likely be charged the price of a pint of the beer, rather than what you've been served, which is half a pint of beer and half a pint of soda.

Drink the first pint as slowly as possible: sip for a while to get the taste, then leave untouched for five to ten minutes before taking bigger gulps.

The speed at which we drink is critical. Especially during the summer, I try to make sure I've drunk a couple of pints of water before I go out, so I'm not drinking for thirst. Otherwise, the first two pints of whatever I drink in the pub will disappear extremely quickly.

It must be possible to train yourself to drink more slowly. I know it's possible to train yourself to drink more quickly because I did it as a teenager. Rich was one of my underage drinking friends and was regarded by all of us with some admiration for the speed at which he downed his beer, as well as his total consumption. One Sunday night in the Bull and Bladder in Brierley Hill, a good thirty-five years ago, I resolved to see how he did it by matching him sip for sip. I was delighted to find that by having a sip every time he had a sip, I could very easily finish a pint as quickly as him. And I never looked back. Slow and steady truly does win the race, I reflected triumphantly.

The question now is how to slow things down a bit, to go back to my rhythm before Rich's quick-sipping Sunday-night masterclass. I occasionally even set the alarm on my watch to go off after, say, three minutes and resolve not to take another sip until it does so.

When I've finished a glass of wine, I find it works well to refill it with water. And pour no more wine into it until I've drunk the water. I tried this with beer once but ended up spending more time in the toilet than at the party.

On what we might call 'round management', Bryn has a modus operandi he's obviously put a lot of thought into:

As your fellow drinkers empty their pint glasses, try to make sure your pint is still a third or a quarter in the glass. On the next round insist on having just a half pint. Ignore the jibes. Toss out some clichés if it helps: 'It's a marathon not a sprint' normally does the trick. When the half is placed in front of you with a scornful snort, pour it into your unfinished pint glass which will then be somewhat full. Continue the sipping/ pausing routine until the next round and repeat as necessary.

As for wine and restaurant drinking, the techniques are similar. I always insist on a small glass. At home I provoke derision from my kids by sipping wine from a sherry glass – but what do they know about drinking?

Gap year

Between school and university I took a gap year. While others travelled the world or knuckled down at work or college, I spent my year at home. By day I worked for my dad's scaffolding company; in the evening I spent my time with that amateur theatre company in Birmingham.

I'd long fancied being an actor but my ambitions had been blunted the year before in the school production of *Cabaret*. The deputy head's husband, an early adopter of new technology, owned a video camera. These were very rare in 1985. He filmed one of the performances and the following week the cast gathered to watch it at school, eager for confirmation of our respective families' verdicts that our performances were quite brilliant. To my dismay it turned out that far from being brilliant in the leading role as a suave but vulnerable American, I was in fact absolutely shit. My accent was more Dudley than Detroit and my singing was dreadful beyond compare.

My dreams of stage and screen hadn't quite died though. I decided a year of am-dram would be the best preparation for taking London theatre by storm when I went off to university there. As ever, regular drinking was part and parcel of the whole enterprise. Most rehearsals ended up, or even took place, in the bar. And after performances, the bar was where you presented yourself to the audience. I tired of trying to gauge what they really thought of my acting, so I just drank instead.

I got to know all manner of different people of different ages from different backgrounds. It was a valuable, enriching experience, which alcohol made all the easier. I don't think I would have got to know these people as well without alcohol to lubricate the machinery of social interaction. I'm not sure if this says something about me, them, or society in general.

Even before my nineteenth birthday, alcohol felt essential to the living of my life. It wasn't so much that I couldn't live without it, or even that I particularly enjoyed it. It was more that I felt, in order to make the most of what came my way, I needed alcohol. People, places and experiences were all better, in my mind, if there was a drink to be taken with them.

I failed to set the world alight in my roles at the Crescent Theatre that year, though I might immodestly claim not to have been entirely dreadful as Derek, the Teddy boy, in Mary O'Malley's *Once A Catholic*. For this part it was suggested I lose a bit of weight. I'm not sure who specified that the Teddy boy should be a skinny Teddy boy, but I was judged to be substantially too portly to squeeze into those drainpipes. To be fair, I was a lumbering mass of fat and muscle. Moving scaffolding about, and eating like a horse, had bulked me up good and proper. I'd have toast before I left home at six in the morning; a humongous breakfast in some transport caff or other at around 9am; fish and chips or some such at lunchtime; dinner back at home and, as often as not, a Balti curry after rehearsals in the evening.

To shift some timber, the director of the production suggested I go on one of those meal replacement milkshake diets for a couple of weeks. 'And no alcohol either,' he said, patting my belly. It says something that the prospect of a fortnight without solid food was less daunting to me than doing without alcohol. Those two dry weeks must have been the longest I'd been without any alcohol in the four years it had taken to become the biggest thing in my young life.

I don't recall particularly struggling to keep off it, but I do vividly remember my first drink after this drought. It was the night before the show opened on the Saturday evening. I was home late after a last rehearsal and treated myself to a small can of lager out of the fridge. Within moments of my first sip, I felt an incredible wave of wellbeing surge through me, flooding my system with the warmest of feelings. I remember thinking, 'Whoa, this alcohol thing really is quite a drug'.

I'm put in mind of a TV advert in which a row of British bobbies, barefoot for some reason, with their trousers rolled up, took sips of Heineken. Such was the power of said lager that it caused their feet to wiggle. Why? Well, 'Heineken Refreshes The Parts Other Beers Cannot Reach', you see. Whatever I was drinking that evening certainly seemed to reach something in me, or so it felt. Or maybe it was merely what that advert, and countless others, had drummed into my young brain that I should be feeling.

Either way, I felt decidedly happy, but shocked at the effect I now saw alcohol had on me. It unsettled me, but also made me love it a little bit more.

🍷🥛🍶

Alcohol was coming in handy with my day job too. Naturally, there was no drinking while I laboured in the yard, drove lorries around, or made a poor job of erecting scaffolding, but it had important uses. I lived a twenty-minute drive away in a different world; a nice, leafy middle-class area where most kids, even then, were expected to go into higher education. My workmates, like all scaffolders, were hard, working men from parts of town I'd only heard about and never visited. I broke bread with many tough guys, some of them ex-prisoners. I saw and heard things I'd not seen or heard before – or since, come to think of it.

Being the boss's son was tricky for me, and for them too. But we got on well, even if we had next to nothing in common apart, of course, from alcohol. To buy a round of beers, and sit around talking, was an insanely effective way of bonding. I drank with them in some of the dodgiest pubs in Birmingham. One Sunday lunchtime, after a weekend scaffolding job, they took me to a pub in Smethwick where, on the sabbath, a stripper was usually to be found performing. I drank a lot, very quickly, as I was wearing tracksuit bottoms and anxious about developing an erection which would have been visible to all. To my relief, the stripper called in sick, so I, along with the rest of this congregation, were spared any embarrassment.

I loved hanging around with this lot. I think they felt the same about me, although this may have been because they thought the boss's son had more money than them and would end up buying most of the drinks. Call me shallow, or naïve, but it still felt good. Taking a couple of lagers with a mixed race lad called Mick in Handsworth; with our erection manager (yes, really) Alan, in the Leather and Bottle in Wednesbury, or with Big Ray, the ex-con, somewhere in Frankley, I felt like I was growing up, pushing back social boundaries as I did so. It was all great.

I was having a tricky but good time at a turning point in my life. Beer seemed to make it less tricky and better all around. Thanks, beer.

Gap-year drinks scorecard

● POSSIBLE INTERVENTIONS

The surge of happiness I'd felt with my first drink following that fortnight's abstinence suggests to me that I was already to some extent addicted. And that in turn suggests that it was already too late for any intervention to make any difference. But why would anyone have bothered anyway? No-one would have thought I needed help, least of all me. I was drinking most days, some more than others, but to no obvious ill effect. I wasn't getting into trouble, be it fighting, drink-driving or having sex. Then again, I was never into fighting or drink-driving anyway, and I still couldn't find anyone to have sex with. My drinking was already where it would be for a good three decades to come, with me putting away much more than was good for me but not enough to raise the alarm bells of anyone who knew me. Not least because the vast majority of them were drinkers rather like me.

● CONSUMPTION

Because I was driving a lot, to work and the theatre, I wasn't drinking quite as much at one sitting, but as I was drinking something most days it was mounting up. If I was driving, I'd push it to a pint and half; when I wasn't driving, I would certainly be drinking – why wouldn't I!? – and drinking more. So, assuming four 'drink-driving' days a week at a pint and a half a pop that's around 14 units. Then I'll throw in a couple of drinking nights with wine and beer which I'd put at eight pints of beer at least and, conservatively, half a bottle of wine – 25 units. And there were odd week nights when I wasn't driving which are probably worth an extra three pints, or seven units. 14 + 25 + 7 gets me to 46 units a week. Let's call the weekly average something **between 40 and 50 units a week**. Incredible. And, just as incredibly, I doubt anyone I was hanging about with at the time considered me a particularly heavy drinker.

● BORING BITS

Few and far between. I still hadn't quite got over the novelty of being able to drink legally. At the theatre and at my dad's scaffolding business I was having a great, if challenging time. However exciting it all was, though, alcohol seemed to make it even better. While a bit of sameness had latterly started to creep into my post-pubescent drinking phase, these new, exciting times stopped the rot.

● PROPORTION OF DRINKS WANTED/ENJOYED/ NEEDED

90 per cent.

14 Units a week? Impossible!

Suggested question for pub quiz: Of all alcohol drinkers in the UK, what percentage drink within the government's recommended safe maximum level? (Answer: somewhere in this chapter.)

Nearly every drinker I know thinks the UK chief medical officers' advice to try to drink no more than 14 units a week is nonsense. They advance many reasons to justify their derision. I believe that I've heard them all. A common one involves a cynical roll of the eyes, accompanied by a sigh and a reminder that, 'It used to be 21 units for men, of course, didn't it? But they changed their minds.' The implication being that the changing of the advice proved it was all a load of nonsense and that 'they' plainly didn't know what they were on about. A bit harsh, that. I'm not sure what else they're supposed to do if the data suggests that the guidance needs changing.

That said, going strictly with the data can lead us into silly places. An example: although the guidance suggests a maximum of 14 units a week for both men and women, the data indicated that drinking even within those guidelines carried with it some risk of harm, especially for women.

This led Dame Sally Davies, then England's Chief Medical Officer, to point out that there was in effect no safe level of drinking. It was at this point that many drinkers, me among them, threw our hands up in despair. On this one I think we might have had a point. Surely, we reasoned, there is no completely safe level of anything.

As David Spiegelhalter, then a Professor for the Public Understanding of Risk, put it:

Given the pleasure presumably associated with moderate drinking, claiming there is no 'safe' level does not seem an argument for abstention. There is no safe level of driving, but the government does not recommend that people avoid driving. Come to think of it, there is no safe level of living, but nobody would recommend abstention.

It was plainly nonsense, and yet more evidence for drinkers like me to conclude that government medical advisers were fanatical killjoys who could safely be ignored.

A better message from the chief medical officers might be something more positive, perhaps pointing out what you could do rather than what you shouldn't be doing. All the focus is on warning about the dangers of drinking more than 14 units a week. A different way of saying the same thing might be to stress that we can drink up to 14 units a week without significant risks to our health.

While I'm sure this would be a better approach, I'll admit that for most drinkers like me it would be irrelevant because, for us, drinking as little as 14 units a week is an absurd idea. We twist our faces in scornful despair and wail, 'But everybody drinks more than 14 units a week.'

The problem is that this simply isn't true.

For a start, there are, believe it or not, people who never go to pubs. During the pandemic lockdown, pubs were shut for months on end. Announcing their mandatory closure at the start of the pandemic, the then-Prime Minister said: 'I do accept that what we're doing is extraordinary: we're taking away the ancient, inalienable right of free-born people of the United Kingdom to go to the pub, and I can understand how people feel about that. It's a huge wrench.'

Heavy stuff this. Ancient? Inalienable? Inseparable from the notion of human freedom itself? I must check the Magna Carta or Domesday Book to find the reference. I happened to watch the Prime Minister's speech in an Irish pub near where I live in West London, and I must admit I nodded along in agreement. Moderate drinker or not these days, I was still assenting to the idea of access to a pub being nothing less than a human right akin to the availability of food and water and somewhere to go to the toilet.

I checked the data on this. It turns out that just over half of adults in England visit pubs, bars or clubs as a free-time activity. This is an awful lot of people, to be sure. But the fact remains that, for more than 20 million adults, licensed premises are an irrelevance, whatever their ancient, inalienable rights might be.

Going back to the data on consumption, nearly ten million people don't drink at all. Of those who do drink, as I've previously said, 5 per cent of all drinkers are putting away vast amounts – more than 50 units, and in many cases well into three figures. And another 25 per cent are drinking between 14 and 50 units a week.

I found this pretty shocking for a while, until I realised that I'd been looking at these numbers through the wrong end of the telescope. I'd been shocked by the wrong thing. The killer fact isn't that 30 per cent of all drinkers are drinking more than 14 units a week; the truly incredible thing, to the minds of drinkers like me anyway, is that *70 per cent of drinkers are managing to drink no more than 14 units a week*. Shockingly, for many of us, moderate, safe drinking isn't the preserve of a handful of light-weights. It's the norm.

Feel free to amaze your friends and infuriate your enemies with this fact. Go on, ask a drinker you know what percentage of their fellow drinkers are drinking within government guide-lines. I have done this countless times, and no-one's ever got anywhere near the correct answer.

When I give them the 70 per cent figure, they generally just refuse to believe it.

If you have a scientific mind, and the time and inclination to read masses of data, by all means come back with the con-clusion that the safe drinking limit is too low. But please don't try and tell me that hardly anybody drinks that little. The fact is that most people who drink, do drink that little. And those of us drinking more than that are the ones in the minority.

🍺 🍷 🍺

As a caveat to all this, I should say that accurate figures on alcohol consumption are notoriously hard to come by. The research largely relies on self-reporting; in other words, it's up to the drinker to record/confess how much they're drinking. Under-reporting is plainly an issue; indeed, by some extrapolations of data on recorded drinking, the amount being consumed is barely half the amount of alcohol being sold. So, unless a lot of it is being put into storage or, even less likely, poured down the drain, something's up. But the data-gatherers are alive to this and make allowances for it.

Even allowing for what would be a grotesquely wide margin of error, I think we can safely say that the 70 per cent figure isn't going to get as low as 50 per cent. So, there's no getting away from it: the majority of drinkers are drinking no more than 14 units a week.

This dirty secret about widespread moderation will stay secret as long as it suits both sides in the argument to keep it that way. Those who campaign on the dangers of excessive drinking focus, naturally enough, on excessive drinking. It hardly suits them to have it out there that most drinkers are drinking safely. They're much more concerned, understandably, with the excessive and dangerous drinking of the minority.

Conversely, you'd have thought the alcohol industry would want to get this happy news of the moderate majority out there, in order to show just what a harmless pastime drinking is for most drinkers. But I suspect the industry is only too keen to have all of us thinking that everyone is drinking too much; that, of course, no-one can manage to drink as little as 14 units a week. The commercial logic being that, if heavy drinkers think everyone else is drinking heavily, they'll feel better about continuing to drink heavily themselves.

The question most drinkers subconsciously ask themselves is: 'If everyone else is doing it, then why shouldn't I?' I know I asked myself this question many times, and always came up with the answer the alcohol companies desired.

This is what psychologists call the 'social norming' of excessive drinking. It's all around us, in every corner of popular culture. It's in the arts, in marketing, advertising, and on just about every greeting card you can buy. Try finding a congratulations card which doesn't feature alcohol.

Drinkers in the 14–50+ unit-a-week category are critically important to the industry. Without us, their profits go down the drain. Just as it's our bracket of drinkers presenting doctors with the most work, it's our group on which the drinks companies are most commercially dependent. If we all moderated to safe levels of drinking, the effect on the industry would be calamitous.

I wish public health specialists would be brave enough to play them at their own game. It's worth a try. How about a poster campaign looking a bit like this:

MOST DRINKERS
DRINK MODERATELY.
BE ONE OF THEM.

or

DO AS MOST
DRINKERS DO:
DRINK SAFELY.

We need to help drinkers like me change the conversations we are having with ourselves. Instead of, *Everyone drinks too much, so why shouldn't I?*, how about *Most people are managing to drink sensibly; so why aren't I?*

University

Having taken a gap year, I was nineteen by the time I got to university in 1986. Westfield College, on the Finchley Road in north-west London, was one of the university's smaller colleges. Unusually for a London college, most of its halls of residence were on-site. My room was a ten-minute walk away in a forbidding building just behind West Hampstead police station. Martyn, he of the beer, roll-ups and heavy rock in his dad's shed, was starting at King's College the same day. Lee, a friend of ours, drove us down to London in a hired van. 'You Can Call Me Al' by Paul Simon will always remind me of that day. Having dropped Martyn off at his halls on Clapham Common, Lee delivered me and my stuff to my decidedly grim-looking new home. 'This looks shit,' he said. And with that he headed back to the West Midlands, quite sure he'd made the right decision in choosing to give university a miss and go into his dad's engineering business instead.

I sat there for a while with a lump in my throat before heading for the college bar – where else? – to try to start making new friends. Up until then, I'd run with the same crowd since the age of four, as we'd all been through the same schools together. We were all drinkers. Now I had to acquire an entirely new friendship group.

In my first week I got to know a lad called Ged, from Consett in County Durham. One day in freshers' week I knocked on his door to see if he was coming to the bar.

'No,' he said. 'I'm off to Mass.'

I laughed; he was a funny guy and I assumed this was one of his deadpan gags. But he was being serious. He said he'd see me in the bar later.

I've always told this tale in the context of religion. I'd never met a Christian who enjoyed beer and football. It was at that moment a journey started which led to my confirmation as a Roman Catholic twenty years later.

But that's another story. What I've come to wondering lately, as I've considered my drinking, is what would have happened if Ged had given me a different answer when I knocked on the door that day and asked if he was coming to the bar. What if he'd said, 'Nah, I don't drink.' The awful truth is that I wouldn't have ended up getting to know him at all. A lifelong friendship would never have happened.

And now I think about it, every one of the many friends I made at college were drinkers. Strange coincidence, that. Oh actually, there was a lad we played football with who never drank, but he was dismissed as a harmless eccentric. Good player, nice lad, bit odd.

And there was a Jordanian medical student called Ali in the room across the hall from me. Fascinating guy, whose dedication to his studies in medicine was matched only by his enthusiasm for the TV show *Blind Date*, on which he made sure to keep me up to date. I asked him once what would happen if, upon qualifying as a doctor, he chose to remain in the UK instead of returning to Jordan. 'They will come and get me,' he said.

He was a decent man who I enjoyed talking to but, as he didn't drink, we were never going to be friends.

Ged, on the other hand, had grown up in a drinking culture at a different level altogether to the one I'd known. Going on a night out with him and his mates in Consett was to witness a level of drinking that made me feel like a novice. They started early and finished late; at no stage was it an option to refuse a pint. One weekend, Martyn the shed man – now an eminent orthodontist, as it happens – came up to Consett with Ged and me. Martyn liked a drink as much as anyone, but not in these quantities. He just about managed to keep up, bless him, until about 1am, by which time we must have been well into double figures. At this point, Martyn cracked. In a tone of quiet desperation I'll never forget, he quietly asked me, as it was my round, if I could get him a bottle of Becks instead of a pint. Not a soft drink, please note, just beer in a smaller vessel.

I snuck it to him when I returned from the bar, but Ged's brother Paddy was on to us in a flash.

'What's your lass drinking?' he demanded.

Martyn's reputation was in tatters; I expect mine was tainted too, merely by association with him. We left town the following morning, under cover of darkness.

Drinking remained central to my university life. I suppose it never occurred to me that it wouldn't, or needn't, have been like that. There are two ways of looking at this. You could say I was already addicted, as alcohol was even then essential to my life. I was in the grip of it before I was out of my second decade. It was a gentle, comforting hold to be sure, but a hold nevertheless. On the other hand, what of it? Let's call the influence alcohol had over me less of a grip than a firm embrace. Rather than squeezing the life out of me, it was helping me squeeze as much fun as possible out of life.

I could have made different choices. I could have chummed up with people who didn't drink, but I never came close to doing so. I wonder how many brilliant people I missed out on. In truth, I probably didn't believe non-drinkers existed.

The fact is, they did. Of course they did. I'm sure I thought that the whole student body was present in the bar at least some of the time; but, considering the size of the bar and the number of us on the campus, the opposite was probably true. Drinkers like me assume everyone else drinks like us. And I suppose I assumed I was only drinking as much as everyone else in my group, but even that might not be true.

Money seemed to be tighter for others than for me so, when I was rounding people up to go to the bar, a few of them would always say they needed to give it a miss as they were short of cash. Three things now strike me about this:

1 No-one, as I recall, ever said they weren't coming because they just didn't want to drink. It was always because they didn't have the money.

2 Very occasionally, someone would say, 'Yeah I'll come, great, but I'm not drinking'. My heart would sink. I'd rather they didn't bother if they'd only be drinking lemonade. I expect that, once we got to the bar, I'd never stop badgering them to have a drink with me.

3 One way or another I'd always find someone who'd drink with me, even just a couple of pints. So it was that I could keep drinking, day after day, week after week, term after term, without thinking I was much different from anyone else. And without anyone else thinking I was drinking more than them.

And I now realise there was another, rather shaming, dynamic in play. It concerns the category of friends I made who were neither non-drinkers, nor big drinkers like me. This group were probably in the majority; they were the ones who didn't mind a drink, even a big drink, every now and then but, unlike me, didn't live their lives by it. These are the ones who I fear I may have helped drag into drinking more. I did so by showing them the pleasure of an afternoon's drinking, or a lock-in, or a wine-box emptying session in someone's room. And it was at these times that I'd be sure to bond with them, perhaps helping turn them into drinkers like me.

Drinkers like me need to do this to normalise our own intake. In doing so, we are brilliant sales reps for the alcohol industry. Not only do we buy lots of their product, we cajole and bully others into doing the same. Brilliant. What a wonderful business model.

I had three objectives for my university life. In order of importance these were as follows: to lose my virginity and go on to have a rich and varied sex life; to drink deeply with a host of new friends; and to be a competent or even brilliant student of English literature. I enjoyed success in only one of these fields. Having lost my cherry in the early hours of a November morning in a house in Cricklewood, I went on to enjoy the sum total of no sexual intercourse whatsoever for the next three and a half years. Long story; let's not go there. I didn't do much better with my studies either. I don't think I ever really got to grips with what I was supposed to be looking for as a student of literature.

When it came to drinking, though, while perhaps not the best of the best, I definitely made the first team. In freshers' week, as is traditional, the student union organised a pub crawl for new boys and girls. I remember turning my nose up at such a thing. It felt to me that such capers weren't for experienced boozers like me. They were more akin to a lacrosse taster session for those who'd never played the game before. No, I didn't need anyone to organise my drinking for me thank you very much. I could do that all on my own. On that night I believe a couple of my new friends and I instead went for a curry, and then got totally pissed in the pub next door and, later, back in the student bar.

Over the next four years as a student, I filled the copious amounts of time I spent neither having sex nor studying, drinking like a man possessed. I shovelled down vast amounts of everything, mostly from heavily scratched reusable plastic glasses in various college bars. And in pubs, student rooms and houses all over London. The craic was mighty, I always tell myself. But when it comes to recalling any particularly brilliant nights, I'm struggling. I definitely remember being quite miserable sometimes, occasionally when I was drinking and often when I wasn't. Incredibly, it's only striking me as I write this, thirty-five years later, that all the drinking may well have been unhelpful vis-à-vis mood – and I doubt it helped me get to grips with girls or books either.

Hang on, though, some good craic is coming back to me:

● One Friday, in my final year, a few of us got involved in an impromptu all-day session in a pub in Kensington. For some reason, three of us saw fit to pop out of the pub late in the afternoon and present ourselves at the ludicrously posh hairdressers around the corner. Here we badgered the poor Frenchman who owned it into shaving each of our heads completely bald. This earned us no small acclaim when we returned to the pub. And when we made it to the college bar for last orders, we got nothing short of a heroes' welcome. Fun for the very feeblest of minds, but what the hell; it's put a smile on my face thirty-one years later.

A friend of mine, Tony, another lad from Consett, still says that one of the funniest things he's ever seen was me, wildly drunk, at two in the morning, standing in the middle of the road outside his college room waving furiously up at him. I had both arms way above my head and a crazy smile on my face. He shouted down at me asking what I was doing. I shouted back that I was trying to wave in the manner of Mary Peters when she was awarded her gold medal in the pentathlon at the 1972 Munich Olympics. The following morning I had only the faintest memory of any of this. And I had no idea at all when it was that I'd seen the footage of the delighted Mary Peters, nor what had given me the notion of doing an impersonation of her for Tony that night. Odd.

Tony, Ged and I – two Geordies and a Brummie – lived with a young man called Paul, who was by some distance the poshest person any of us had ever come across. He was tremendously tall with perfect, pure skin. His manners were exemplary. He could talk to anyone and was game for anything. And, of course, he liked a drink. I loved him; we all loved him.

He took me to Twickenham to see England play Wales at rugby; I took him to various West Brom matches. Possessing a fine singing voice, honed in his school choir, he'd join in the terrace chanting with great gusto. The operatic timbre of his voice attracted one or two quizzical glances from my fellow West Brom fans. 'West Brom aggro; West Brom aggro. Hello!' he'd boom, pronouncing the 'hello' as he would have done in greeting a village vicar cycling past.

One time, standing in the Birmingham Road End at a particularly dismal home game, a derisive chant started up, aimed at our soon to be sacked manager, Ron Saunders. Pardon my language here, but it went like this:

Saunders is a cunt, Saunders is a cunt
The Brummie Road will sing this song
Saunders is a cunt.

Always quick to pick out a tune and lyrics, Paul weighed in with his rich baritone. After a couple of minutes, as the chant died away, he tapped me on the shoulder and asked, 'Who's Saunders?'

Another time I took my man to see West Brom play at Grimsby Town. We went on the train and drank an awful lot. In Cleethorpes, where Grimsby's ground is, we carried on drinking. He was wearing a long tweed overcoat accessorised with a West Brom scarf I'd given him. We sank beers as we chatted with various West Brom fans of my acquaintance. They stared at him in wonder, like they might observe giraffes or zebras at West Midlands Safari Park. They'd never met the like. When he went for a wee, someone said, 'Where the fook you find him, Ade?'

Walking into the ground, the two of us were pulled aside by a policeman who pointed out, correctly, that we'd plainly had a vast amount to drink and should watch our step. 'Absolutely, officer,' bellowed my fabulously posh friend. 'Many apologies sir.' The copper looked puzzled and waved us on. We staggered up on to the terrace in the away end to watch West Brom score early but then lose. We slept all the way back to London. It was a magnificent day. My friend is now a judge and is addressed as His Honour. He still enjoys a pint.

Sometimes the drinking was all great fun; sometimes the drinking was boring. But I was always drinking. A bit of boorishness crept in from time to time – singing and general horseplay on public transport, that kind of thing. I don't think I caused much harm to anyone apart from, arguably, myself. What's for sure is that university reinforced a state of mind I'd spent my teens drinking my way into: the stone-cold certainty that the prospect of life – or even so much as a night out – was quite impossible to relish without alcohol being taken.

Shortly after I left, Westfield College in Hampstead was closed down and merged with Queen Mary College in the East End of London. The Hampstead land was sold for redevelopment. On it now stands a collection of eyewateringly expensive residences. When I'm in that area I occasionally stop by for a wander around. I consider the significant traces of alcohol to be found in the soil beneath these penthouses, like chemical waste on brownfield sites in less salubrious parts of town.

Having finished my final exams in the spring of 1990, I devoted myself to watching football's World Cup. For England's semi-final against Germany a load of us gathered at my flat. Naturally, there was drinking involved. In fact, looking back, the evening was as much about alcohol as football. We could hardly have been more excited in the build-up but must have felt the need to enhance that excitement by drinking an enormous amount before kick-off. During the match itself, alcohol was deployed to quell our nerves and ease the anxiety. After England lost to penalties, we addressed our misery with yet more alcohol. Those of us still capable of speech talked about our feelings of emptiness now that we were out of the tournament and had to face up to the fact that our student life was over, and the big, wide world beckoned. We carried on drinking.

In the morning, calamitously hungover, I asked myself what on earth I was going to do with the rest of my life. I had no answer. For want of anything else to do, I got a job at a summer school in Rickmansworth teaching English to teenagers from elsewhere in Europe. As ever, I gravitated towards the drinkers among the other teachers, and indeed some students, and continued to drink deeply and regularly. I had idle thoughts about staying in academia. My tutor had said I could possibly be looking at a first-class degree. I was sitting in a pub in Rickmansworth when the tutor called me to say that the first-class degree had not, as it turned out, materialised. Neither for that matter, had a 2:1. I was most disappointed, not to say devastated, to hear that I'd been awarded a 2:2. I was even more devastated that my tutor didn't seem to share my astonishment; what she'd said about me getting a first had apparently slipped her mind. Perhaps I'd dreamt it.

🍷 🥃 🍺

I resolved to qualify as a teacher of English as a foreign language, and then find a teaching job in Croatia. The course took place in October, just off Piccadilly in London. My fellow students were a mixed bag of new graduates and the middle-aged. All of us seemed vaguely lost. I identified the drinkers in the group, and we overshared life stories in the pubs of Shepherds Market. Great nights, great conversations. I was still of the opinion that these evenings could only happen with the assistance of alcohol. I often still think that.

Halfway through the course I smashed my left leg in two playing football. I needed an operation to wangle the bones back together. I told the anaesthetist about a bad experience I'd had with a previous general anaesthetic. She gave me what she called an 'especially generous' pre-med to calm me down. In went that jab and before long this cocktail of Valium and who knows what else was working its magic.

Here I was, alone in a hospital in Hemel Hempstead, leg smashed and nascent teaching career in jeopardy, feeling absolutely terrific about a world of possibilities opening up in front of me. Remarkable. I mention this because the only experience I could compare to the feeling that injection gave me was that first drink I had after two weeks not drinking in preparation for the play I did in my gap year. That's how powerful the pre-med was. That's how powerful alcohol is.

Soon, of course, misery prevailed again as I came around after the operation with a giant cast on my leg and absolutely no idea what lay ahead. I asked the doctor if a post-med was available as strong as the pre-med. He shook his head.

Before the accident, to my delight, I'd had a tenuous offer of a job teaching English at the British Council in Zagreb. This now evaporated as, although I managed to finish my course and secure the qualification, it was seven months before I shed that cast, and twelve months before I could walk properly. I went back to live with my parents for a year, eating and drinking an enormous amount. I still managed to get to the pub most nights. When it snowed that winter, a friend of mine who is now a doctor towed me there on a sledge.

By the time I got off my crutches they might have been bowed from supporting my now huge weight; sitting around drinking and eating without doing any exercise at all had predictable consequences. With the teaching post in Zagreb having faded away, I managed to get on a journalism course at the Cardiff Institute of Higher Education. There I worked diligently on acquiring knowledge on matters pertaining to journalism and increasing still further my intake of alcohol. I didn't know if I'd find gainful employment anywhere as a journalist. I suppose I must have assumed that if I did, my flair for drinking would be every bit as useful as my shorthand or rudimentary knowledge of media law.

University drinks scorecard

● POSSIBLE INTERVENTIONS

How could these years have been different? Looking back, at these and other phases of my drinking life, I always end up identifying hypothetical people I could have encountered in my life who might have changed things, or, rather, changed me. But I'm aware there is room to blame myself too; I could have made different choices all on my own. That would have been hard though, given that society – at least the bits I knew – seemed to be encouraging me to drink deeply every step of the way.

I sense that by now it would have taken something as dramatic as the influence of, say, a religious sect to have changed my direction. Perhaps I could have been convinced that the devil himself would come and take me for his own if I didn't stop drinking the thirty-odd pints of ale I was putting away every week.

● CONSUMPTION

Drinking had definitely become a habit by now; a constant, almost like eating or going to the toilet. I doubt I had more than two days off a week and the other five would certainly have involved some pretty spectacular sessions, at least three a week. On these sessions I reckon I had at least eight pints of beer, or the equivalent in wine. Eight pints come in at around 20 units, so that's 60 a week for starters. On the other nights I'd be looking at two pints at the very least so that's another 8 units. 68 units in total is a hell of a big number but I've got to say I think it's the lowest number

I can get to with a straight face. Let's call it somewhere **between 65 and 80 units a week**. Ye gods. And I must stress again that I was not considered by any means a huge drinker.

● BORING BITS

Night after night chugging back beer.

Staying up half the night talking shite, before staggering to bed in the early hours having had not much fun at all.

And so on.

● PROPORTION OF DRINKS WANTED/NEEDED/ENJOYED

60 per cent.

Her name is Llana and she is a moderator

Llana Harkins, mid-thirties, has always worked in sales and lives in the Glasgow area. Our second moderator, she used to drink loads, but now hardly at all.

I started drinking when I was fifteen. I was always like a party animal. Even when I was in my twenties, I was clubbing all weekend. And then I had kids – I had my son at 29 – and I feel like my drinking definitely improved. But there were still the special nights I was having with my friends, when I'd just revert back to my old habits, and it started to have an impact on my mental health.

So, on average I suppose it'd be about a bottle of prosecco on a Friday and a Saturday night. Perhaps a couple of glasses of wine on a Thursday, and maybe the same on a Sunday.

But if I went on a proper night out, I'd drink an obscene amount. I drank maybe like gin and tonic or something else, which I am normally fine on. But then, as soon as I got out – you know the feeling before you've even left the house; it's your old self. You're full of excitement and anxiety and you're off.

Talking to Llana, it's clear she can still feel what that excitement and – interesting word – *anxiety* felt like. Yet she's in a different place entirely now.

I did try moderating my drinking, but I would always get carried away and I just couldn't shake that. So I stopped completely. A couple of things happened: my brother went into rehab for his cocaine problem. I saw him sober and thought I could do it too. Then I was out one night and drank so much I blacked out. I thought, right that's enough.

And so the drinking stopped completely for fifteen months.

I just thought, life's gonna be so boring; what will I do? How is it gonna affect my friendships, and my relationship as well, because my partner and I drank a lot together. But very quickly I realised that life was so much better. And the mental health aspect was very real. I definitely suffered from anxiety after drinking so that just went away.

If life was so much better without alcohol, then why start drinking again at all? All moderators, at some point, are asked this. Llana's answer is interesting.

I realised that for me to stay sober I had to really be very sort of anti-alcohol, which didn't really feel that peaceful. I saw I had to in a way try to make peace with alcohol.

Believers in 'alcoholism' as a 'disease' might well contest the very idea of 'making peace' with alcohol. I find the notion fascinating. You obviously can't be at peace with drinking if it has you in its control, if you're drinking way more than is good for you and paying a price for it. But neither, Llana reasons, can you be at peace with it (or yourself, really) if you're so 'against' it that you're not touching a drop. That would make her feel as if she was still in some sense at war with it; as if there was unfinished business.

I just got curious about whether or not I am a person that could moderate and take it or leave it with just like one drink, you know, in social circumstances when other people are drinking. I think I wanted to show it was possible because I think it's the prospect of completely stopping drinking that puts people off dealing with their alcohol issues in the first place. A lot of people just can't compute the idea of sobriety forever.

It wasn't as if I just fell back into it. I thought about it long and hard; I had a very well thought-out strategy in place before I started drinking again. I don't think I fell off the wagon; with that plan in place, I felt like I dismounted gracefully.

'Dismounted gracefully' from the wagon. My moderators all seem to have a lovely way with words.

So, my strategy now that I'm back drinking: I don't drink high ABV drinks. I'll either drink like a low alcohol beer, or I'll have a beer with the lowest ABV. I researched what had the fewest units and saw that it was maybe a gin and tonic, so I'll have that. I always use a measure; I don't do 'home measures' or anything anymore. I'll always have lots of tonic. And I'm aware now of just enjoying it more and I'm not looking for an effect, if you know what I mean. I don't think I've even been tipsy since I started drinking again, and I've certainly not been drunk.

And I don't drink at all if I don't feel good. But also, I don't drink if I have that Friday feeling, because I know how that ends and it's not good. As I'm already on a high I just enjoy that high and don't drink on top of it. That might sound weird.

Well at first it does sound weird, I suppose, until you realise it's a perfectly logical point. I get more of an urge to drink when I'm feeling happy, celebrating good things, rather than when I'm down, lamenting bad things. I've always congratulated myself for generally being sensible enough not to drink when I'm feeling down. Not for the first time in this drinking caper have I now realised that I needed to ask myself a different question: why the need to drink when I'm happy? Why not take the Llana approach instead and, when I'm feeling good, just enjoy that feeling instead of using alcohol to try to augment it? Mad.

I definitely needed the break because I had to learn how to socialise better. I had to build my confidence and my self-esteem; I had to get good coping strategies. It will always be the best thing I've ever done for myself because now I have my self-esteem, and I'm so much more confident than I used to be. And there's so much more to life now. Before I stopped, I just felt is this it? Is this all my life's about? I realise that drinking for me was just lazy fun, that's what it was for me.

Lazy fun. Yes, that's right: it's the laziest, easiest way to have something you convince yourself is fun. And I suppose you could argue there's not a lot wrong with that, to which Llana would say, you can have much more fun if you work harder at it.

I didn't have to think what I wanted to do to have fun; I'd just open a bottle of prosecco and that would be it. Now I go hillwalking and wakeboarding and all sorts of things. I think of all the time I used to give to drinking instead of doing these things. And now I feel I have life in technicolour; I really feel that way.

These days Llana barely drinks at all.

I might have maybe two or three drinks a month. The most I've had in one go was three, but that was over nine hours when some friends came over. Sometimes I just have an alcohol-free beer. I really don't need it anymore.

For some people, moderating is about squeezing as much enjoyment – lazy fun, if you like – out of alcohol as they can. For Llana, it seems rather different. She's so 'over' drinking that it hardly matters to her whether she's drinking or not. She has no love or appetite for it anymore but, importantly for her, neither does she hate it. By stopping completely, and then coming back to it on her own terms, she's made her peace with it. I suspect she would never have felt this way had she remained completely abstinent.

Why the health warnings don't apply to me

Look, I know I drink more than I'm supposed to, but I don't think it's a problem for me because it's mostly red wine I drink; that's quite good for you, isn't it?

There are plenty of things you can say to convince yourself that the advice on safe levels of alcohol intake doesn't apply to you. There's so much data about now, on just about any subject you care to name, that there's bound to be some evidence somewhere to support or undermine just about any proposition you care to make. Seek and you shall find. The trouble is that most of us don't bother to read the actual research, or even a newspaper story about it, especially if the headline is to your liking.

A classic example of this is the idea that red wine is good for you. The evidence suggests, as I understand it, that red wine has some health benefits which may outweigh the harm the alcohol is doing, but only if the red wine is taken in small quantities (certainly no more than the official suggested maximum of

14 units a week). Unhelpfully though, in media coverage of this story, words like 'moderate' and 'glass or two' are used, which are essentially meaningless unless defined. Even more unhelpful is the attention-grabbing, newspaper-selling, click-generating headline which will reduce the whole thing down to 'RED WINE IS GOOD FOR YOU'. Before you know it you're thinking of red wine as a health drink, perhaps even counting towards one of your five-a-day fruits or vegetables.

There's so much material to work with here. As well as the medical evidence you choose to believe in, there will be old wives' tales, stuff a mate told you once, and ideas you subscribe to without knowing where you got them from. Maybe you heard something you wanted to hear on the radio, or from someone in the pub who'd heard it from someone who'd heard it from a doctor.

Here are some very common ones I've heard many times, not least from the voice in my own head.

Look, I know I drink more than I'm supposed to, but I don't think it's a problem for me because ...

... I'm a big bloke
... who wants to live forever anyway?
... everything's bad for you, according to them.
... I drink lots of water.
... whatever you drink just flushes through you, so what's the problem?
... Guinness is good for you.
... .er, what's a unit again?
... I do a lot of exercise so that just sweats it all out.
... I have lots of days off which gives my body a chance to recover.

... I just get completely smashed twice a week and otherwise don't drink.

... I don't binge; I just drink a little every day.

... the doctors know nothing.

... my grandad/uncle/aunt/neighbour/friend drank a bottle of whisky a day and lived to be 80.

... I feel fine.

... I know for a fact my doctor drinks more than I do.

... I don't get hangovers so it can't be doing me much harm.

... it's the nanny state gone mad.

... lots of people drink stacks more than me and they're doing OK.

... if I didn't drink, I'd be unhappy and that would make me ill.

It's amazing how much tosh we can believe if we want to.

Underage again

The summer after my first year at university I went off to America. A couple of friends and I flew to Los Angeles and, six weeks later, back from New York. In between we travelled from west to east coast on Greyhound buses. Big Jim and Chops (nicknames; long story) were friends from home and both older than me, 22 and 23 respectively. I was only just twenty. I knew the minimum drinking age in the States was twenty-one but assumed I was close enough to get away with it. To my dismay it turned out that American doormen and bar staff adhered to their minimum age rules a lot more closely than their British cousins.

On our first evening in Los Angeles, I elicited shakes from a bartender's head everywhere we tried. We ended up in some cheap Chinese restaurant where my mates, randomly as you like, spotted those odd-looking blokes from the pop duo Sparks. They were excited beyond measure. I just sat there miserably. The old dread anxiety about getting served alcohol, which I thought I'd left behind on my eighteenth birthday more than two years earlier, came flooding back.

So here I was, about to embark on the coast-to-coast trip of a lifetime, thinking only of how crap it was going to be if I couldn't drink whenever it pleased me to do so. I carried this anxiety, by bus, from LA to Santa Barbara and San Francisco; on to Salt Lake City, Austin, New Orleans, Atlanta, North Carolina, Philadelphia, and New York. Upon arrival in each city, the only thing on my mind was whether or not we'd find somewhere to go where I'd be served alcohol. Sometimes we found somewhere; sometimes we didn't.

Don't get me wrong; this didn't mar the entire experience. It was still the trip of a lifetime but, looking back, through the prism of the bottom of a glass, two things shock me. Firstly, how crazy and sad it is that for nearly four and a half thousand miles the question of where and when I was going to be served my next drink was never far from my mind.

Secondly, when I sift through my precious memories of that summer, the clearest and happiest of them all involve alcohol.

There was an epic afternoon's drinking in a bar in Santa Barbara where some nice gay men became fascinated by us and our Black Country accents.

In San Francisco there were some girls I vaguely knew from college in London who were studying at Berkeley for a year. We met up with them and drank lots of wine in their dorms.

In Salt Lake City a drink wasn't to be had anywhere, but I did visit an all-you-can-eat restaurant for the first time in my life. I ate so much that the kitchen staff came out to have a look at me.

Austin was great. I always said it was my favourite stop, and it was. But I suspect my fondness for the place was mainly because, for some reason, I was able to drink with impunity there.

In Chapel Hill, North Carolina, Jim had a friend from home who was doing a PhD there, so he could pull some strings. We had a mad, bad, great night.

And in Philadelphia there was a ballet dancer called Mina who I'd very much taken a shine to when I'd met her through a mutual friend the year before in the UK. We arranged to meet

135

her, but she disappointed me greatly by turning up with a bloke called Jimmy. I was disconsolate but, on a more positive note, they'd chosen a restaurant where they were happy to serve me alcohol, so the edge was taken off my dismay. For dessert, Mina ate something featuring blackberries, little bits of which, unknown to her, remained stuck in her teeth. Jim whispered to me, 'Mina, Mina – her teeth could be cleaner.' He knew how to cheer me up, that Jim – still does. Alcohol plus daft humour works every time. We all had a nice enough evening in the end.

Mina popped into my mind a couple of years ago. I found her on the internet running a dance project somewhere on the east coast. I sent her a nice email. She replied saying, 'I remember your name, but your face not at all.' I can't have made much of an impression on her.

Should I be grateful that alcohol made these nights possible and/or bearable, or worry that I already felt I so desperately needed a drink to have a good time, or at least to not have a bad time?

Underage US-road trip drinks scorecard

● POSSIBLE INTERVENTIONS
If my friends on that trip hadn't been drinkers too, then maybe it would all have been different. But if they hadn't been drinkers, I doubt I would have been friends with them anyway.

● CONSUMPTION
I couldn't drink every day, so that would have brought my numbers down a bit. Naturally, when I did get the chance to drink, I drank as much as I possibly could. Let's say there were a dozen proper drinking nights over the six weeks we

were away, at each of which I suppose the equivalent of six pints were sunk. So let's call it six pints multiplied by twelve sessions which comes to 72 pints. Per week that's around twelve pints which would have been **less than 30 units**.

● PROPORTION OF DRINKS WANTED/NEEDED/ENJOYED

100 per cent. With supply of it restricted, every drink was worth more. Less was more. Interesting. This was, I suppose, what I've now come to know as mindful drinking. While it's significant, not to say disappointing, that alcohol was already so central to my enjoyment of life, this episode also illustrates the power of drinking less. If access to alcohol had been unrestricted, I would have drunk more and enjoyed it less.

Moderation is hard

I recently went on a retreat, in Australia. It's not my kind of thing but my wife talked me into it. In its favour were the surroundings; up in untamed hills looking down upon the Gold Coast we would be living in some comfort. On the downside was the prospect of a whole week without alcohol, sugar, gluten, dairy or coffee. In between not enjoying these things we would be exercising in a range of strenuous and/or mindful ways. Also on offer would be therapies and treatments for various maladies, real and imagined, and lectures on what was good and bad for you to eat, do, drink and think. Each day began with a smart rap on the door of our quarters at 5.45. This was our signal to get out of bed and assemble for a quick burst of qigong on the side of a hill. In the gentlest possible way, this was hardcore.

I dreaded most of this but ended up loving nearly all of it. The highlights included sessions by an ex-hurdler on joint flexibility; a softly spoken lady who taught us how to brutalise ourselves with a foam roller; and an hour of horse therapy in which, despite every effort on my part to resist, I became very emotional with an old horse called Bono. As for the lowlights, I won't be in a hurry to have my colon irrigated again any time soon, and I can't say I much enjoyed a stomach massage executed by a large woman from Brisbane who dotted her patter with lots of political opinions I disagreed with.

Breakfast, lunch and dinner, all astoundingly delicious, were served at the same time each day; we ate at tables of eight, with the seating plan changing from meal to meal as, with algorithmic precision, we were shuffled so that every inmate got to break (gluten free) bread with every other inmate at least once over the course of a week. Most mealtimes I tried to beat the system to inveigle myself onto a table with a macho cattle station owner called Bruce, who I found fascinating company. The nearest shop to his home on the station in north Queensland was an hour away, by air. I'd think how much I'd have loved a couple of pints with this chap.

The whole experience taught me three valuable lessons:

● Firstly, for a week at least and probably longer, I can manage without dairy, sugar or gluten. I was fine without alcohol too. Since there was none available I didn't feel as if I was missing out. And, interestingly, it was a blessed relief not to bother thinking about it for a week. How much time and energy I must regularly expend on planning my next drink, or how not to drink.

Coffee, though, was a different matter. Many of my fellow retreaters were in a similar boat, most of them reporting searing headaches. I didn't get headaches, but for forty-eight hours I might as well have been in bed with a migraine for all the use I was. I quite literally could not stay awake. If I was eating or exercising, I could just about keep my eyes open; but as soon as I stopped moving, I conked out. By day three, though, the fug cleared and I felt great. Another blessed relief.

● Secondly, while I didn't miss alcohol, I did wonder how different it would have been if there had been alcohol allowed and a bar for us to enjoy a drink together. Without the benefit of alcohol, I had some good conversations with some interesting people, but I wonder if there would have been more of these if drinks could have been taken. This could well be merely what my alcohol-dependent brain is telling me, but I imagine that after dinner every evening a few of us would have repaired to the bar and ended up talking long into the night. The craic would have been good. In the morning at qigong, knowing smirks would have been exchanged. As it was, none of that happened. Instead, we said our good nights at about 8.30. In the absence of booze, several great bonds of friendship may not have been forged. But that was a small price to pay to be able to sleep the sleep of the virtuous until the dawn qigong wake-up call bore down on us again.

● Thirdly, and most importantly, while I learned a lot about dairy, coffee, sugar, gluten and alcohol, none of it would prove very useful in the long run because everything was geared to total abstinence. Yes, we realised we felt better for not touching any of the above. We understood why. But in our real lives this probably wouldn't be practical for us to achieve. It would have been really good to get some guidance about how to moderate our usual intake. But, among all the interesting and informative talks we were given, not one minute was spent on the biggest challenge we were all to face the moment we walked out of the camp gates at the end of the week: how to cut down on the bad-for-you-five of coffee, sugar, dairy, gluten and booze. Not a word about useful strategies to cut down on any of them. Staying off these things for a week was the easy bit; staying off them once we were back in our normal lives, with no qigong dawn calls, would be a different matter. How to moderate our intake was the biggest question that needed answering, and no time whatsoever was devoted to it.

Moderation, especially with alcohol, is nobody's friend. If you cut your drinking down, big boozers and teetotallers alike will be unimpressed.

🍷 🥤 🍺

Safe, moderate drinking. Even as I write those words, part of me stifles a yawn. I get that; not as much as I did when I was really tanking it, but I still get it. I've thought it for so long that it's difficult to stop thinking it. The very point of most drugs, after all, is to lose yourself a bit by altering something going on in your brain. And if a job's worth doing, I suppose the logic goes, it's worth doing properly. This is one reason it's hard to moderate. There are many others.

The English language itself seems to conspire against moderation. There are very few words to describe the feeling you get when you've had a few, safe, moderate drinks. I could only think of five, and two of those I'd never heard of before my teenage daughters suggested them.

Merry
Tipsy
Wavey
Tiddly
Buzzed

Compare and contrast the words available to describe your condition after an unsafe, immoderate amount to drink:

Drunk
Blind drunk
Rolling drunk
Well-oiled

Hammered
Rat-arsed
Ratted
Fucked
Sozzled
Tanked up
Pissed
Pissed out of your head
Pissed out of your mind
Pissed as a fart
Pissed as a newt
Smashed
Stramashed
Wankered
Shitfaced
Mortal
Steaming
Out of it
Trollied
Sloshed
Gone
Spangled
Bladdered
Off your face
Jam crackered

Note how many of these words imply that harm is being done.

I know that stopping drinking completely isn't easy, but complete abstinence does have at least one clear advantage over moderation: it involves taking one decision, and one decision only. Whether you can stick to it or not is a different matter; the important thing is that everyone knows what it is that you are trying to do. I've gone without alcohol completely for long stretches; well, Lent anyway. And when you're used to drinking something every day, the forty-six days and nights of Lent without a drop can feel like a life sentence. But it still felt simpler than cutting down. Everybody knew I was off drinking, so I wasn't pressed into it, by me or anyone else.

In contrast, if you choose instead to moderate, things are less clear. That one decision you've made to drink less isn't the only one you'll have to make. Far from it. Dozens more lie ahead of you; there'll be many to make most days. You'll have to decide when to drink or not drink. Only at weekends? Every other weekend? One day every weekend? The choice is yours. Then there's what to drink, how much of it to drink, when to start drinking it and when to stop. You also have to decide who to drink with. This last one can be the most difficult call of all. Alcohol is the only drug you need to apologise for not taking.

If I decide to drink with old friend number one, that's fine. But if, a couple of days later, I meet old friend number two on a night I'm not drinking, or perhaps just drinking a little, what if I mention the big night out I had a couple of days earlier with friend number one? It's not inconceivable that friend number two will be miffed. I know I've been miffed by this kind of thing in my time. This is what happens when the circle of friends you've assembled around you all happen to be drinkers like you.

Let's say you meet one of your friends, someone you'd normally share a bottle of wine with, and you don't get to see them that often. What do you do? There are so many options, many of which feel decidedly sub-optimal. You could try covertly drinking less than they do, and hope they make up the difference. Or you could say you'll 'just have a glass'. This may well annoy your friend. Do they order the bottle and drink more of it, or buy it by the glass, which gets expensive? Alternatively, you could not drink wine at all and go for something different. Or tellingly, it might just be simpler to say you're not drinking at all because you're on antibiotics or something. Whatever you do, if drinking with this friend is what you've always done and looked forward to doing, there's a real possibility you'll offend them.

If I'm meeting a good friend who I've not seen for a while, there'll generally be an expectation that we drink together because that's what we've always done and is, I'm afraid, part of the bond between us.

A friend I'd not seen for a while turned up to meet me in a pub a couple of years ago. As I made for the bar he said, 'I'll just have a half; I'm driving.' Those were the actual words he used, but what it felt like he'd said was, 'I'll just have a half; you don't mean so much to me as a friend anymore.' Honestly, I felt hurt. Ludicrous. We sat in this pub, had a meal, during which he drank two halves of weak bitter, and I didn't have much more. It was really great to catch up; a lovely evening. On the long journey home on the tube, I reflected on the lesson learned: it's fine not to drink much; our friendship didn't actually depend on it after all.

But if he pulled the same trick again next time, there would be trouble. He didn't, thankfully. Good sense prevailed and we went back to drinking lots when we met, and having a nice time, though not any nicer than when we hardly drank much at all. Old habits die hard.

The social pressure we put each other under to drink is intense. If I've been cooking all day for some friends coming around for dinner, woe betide anyone who turns up not planning to honour my efforts by drinking with me. Driving? 'What do you mean you're driving? I've not stopped since ten o'clock this morning and this is the thanks I get!' I've thought this several times and said it out loud more than once.

This nonsense had to stop. After I finished making my TV documentary, I made a solemn promise to myself: I would never again pressure anyone into drinking a drop more than they wanted to, and neither would I take it personally if they weren't drinking when I would have expected them to do so. And I also swore that I'd never allow myself to be pressurised by anyone else into drinking more than I wanted, whatever offence, consternation or disappointment this caused.

A few weeks later I was working away in Manchester. Every now and then I'd get together with a colleague called Rebecca for a few drinks. We hadn't met up for a while so along she came to meet me in the bar in my hotel, which was our usual routine before heading off somewhere to eat. I asked her what she was drinking, and, to my suppressed disappointment, she asked for a mineral water as she said she was driving. Breezily, for all the world as if I was totally cool with this, I got beer for me and water for her.

I told her about my pledge not to pressure anyone to drink but, as the evening progressed, I found myself gently badgering her to have a small one, and even possibly leave her car in the hotel car park and so on. In the end, with good-natured exasperation, she said, 'Adrian, I'd love a drink, but I'm pregnant.' I felt a complete buffoon. Rebecca and her husband now have a toddler, and I look forward to toasting all their good health with them soon. And if they're not drinking that evening that's fine. Obviously, it's just fine.

I think I have now changed my ways. I won't pressure anyone to drink; I won't be pressured by anyone. I used to drink getting on for 100 units every week; now I drink less than a third of that. And I still enjoy drinking. Some achievement, I'm sure you'll agree, so where's my medal? There isn't one, because us moderators are so scandalously uncelebrated. Heavy drinkers don't like us because we're lightweights and/or shine a light on their own shortcomings. Abstainers don't like us because they think we're in denial about our issues and should really be giving up completely like them. We moderators must plough on regardless; our achievements largely unrecognised, uncelebrated and even scorned.

Twenties

Every other drinking memoir you'll ever read will reach a point when everything falls apart. There will be a terrible accident, chronic illness, appalling misbehaviour, destitution, or some other drama. Allow me to manage your expectations: this is not what happened in my case. I just drank more and more without any immediately apparent harm visited on myself or anyone else. That's kind of the point; it's precisely why drinkers like me are so imperilled. We don't get the warning signs.

It wasn't my intention to trawl through my drinking life story, because on the face of it, there wasn't a lot to say. It all felt terribly mundane, but I'm glad I took the trouble, if only for my own benefit. Or at least I think I'm glad I did. I've been shocked to realise quite how much I was drinking and for how long. I've often said that my life has revolved around alcohol, but it's only now I see just how dreadfully true that has been for an awful long time. From the very first sips onwards, I can see how the seeds were sown and how they've grown.

My first day at the BBC, on work experience, naturally concluded with an evening in the pub, as did the vast majority of the days of my working life thereafter. My boss then, to whom

I owe pretty much everything career-wise, was a brilliant, maverick television man called Paul Gibbs. Many hearts were broken when he died from cancer in his early sixties. Paul loved life, loved a drink and apparently loved me. Naturally, these things all commended him to me. It was the happiest of times. I'd found the kind of work I wanted to be in, and I was surrounded by great people who taught me a huge amount and, in most cases, drank a huge amount too.

In the old days, from what I'm told, television newsrooms amounted to pubs in which typewriters, computers and the odd TV screen were the only clues that television was made there. Now it's entirely different. I think it's fair to say that our office, where we made a show called *Business Breakfast*, was one of the last to change. Drinks trollies, clinking with promise, were forever being wheeled in; replenishment of the fridge in Paul's office was taken very seriously. As we were working on an early morning programme, we were done and dusted by 9am. A couple of glasses of something or other were generally supped after a night shift.

I was initially in Paul's department for just three weeks of work experience. Not knowing my arse from my elbow about business news or television production, there wasn't an awful lot I could usefully do, so I just resolved to make myself indispensable in any way I could think of. This turned out to be relatively easy. I ran the odd journalistic errand, but mainly supplied tea and coffee on demand and made myself available to anyone who needed a drinking companion any time of day or night. At the end of my three weeks, I was offered a contract as a production assistant.

I'm not saying it was only my enthusiasm for drinking that led to the bonding that led to the job, but it did no harm. One of the first friends I made was the journalist and presenter, Adam Shaw, with whom I went on to work for many years. He wasn't a massive drinker, and neither did he have any interest in football. I mention this as he once said how he envied me my interest in football because, on all sorts of social occasions and work trips he'd see how football was an instant conversation point for me; a really useful social lubricant not available to him. He's right about the football, and I suspect the same applies to drinking. How to win friends and influence people? Drink with them! I wonder now if those three weeks' work experience would have led to a job, and a long career in the business, if I hadn't been a drinker. I honestly don't think they would. It's not that Paul picked me for my boozing; rather that I can't think of any other way I could have got the time with him to get to know him and enable him to form any kind of opinion of me at all.

The short contract led to a full-time job. I was the happiest man alive. There was a two-month gap before the job started in earnest, so I decided to go on an adventure. I bought a decent bicycle, loaded it up with as much clobber as I could carry, and cycled to Croatia.

🍷 🥃 🍺

This was 1992 and Yugoslavia was at war with itself. My odyssey was part a gesture of solidarity, and part weight-loss measure. The two stone I'd put on while incapacitated with my broken leg needed shifting. I got the ferry overnight to Hamburg and ped-alled from there to Berlin and on to Prague, Vienna, Bratislava, Budapest and Zagreb.

On my first night, shattered after the furthest I'd ever cycled in one go, I stayed in Lüneberg. I had a beer in a bar and fell into conversation with a local. I told him what I was up to. 'Ah!' he exclaimed. 'A ride for peace!' I said I hadn't thought about it like that, but now he mentioned it, why not? To show his support, he bought my beer all evening.

I drank every night of that trip. It never occurred to me not to. It's only thirty years on that it's dawned on me how extraordinary it is that this was my normal. Alone, usually, in bars and restaurants across Eastern Europe, I'd drink a little or a lot, but always something. If I found a bit of company, so much the better.

In the Czech border town of Dečín I fell in with another cyclist for a couple of days, a retired dentist from Kansas called Jerome J. Mindrup, who sounded like Jimmy Stewart. We clinked glasses, exchanged life stories, and drank nicely together.

In Prague I was in the company of a distant friend of a distant friend, a young woman called Romana, whose mum fed me lavishly. Disastrously though, neither of them drank. But to my delight and relief I ran into a big group of blokes from Edinburgh, fans of Heart of Midlothian, who were there to play Slavia Prague. That was my drinking sorted, good and proper.

One night in a restaurant in the middle of nowhere in Slovakia, I was so engrossed in whatever I was reading that I lost track of how much wine I'd drunk. When I stood up, everything was swimming a bit. Adding to my confusion, this rural restaurant was suddenly full of African men. They turned out to be Angolans taking part in some kind of socialist brotherhood exchange. I closed my book, sobered up a bit, and focussed on drinking a whole lot more with my new Angolan friends.

All great times. Great experiences with great people. And, less by luck than judgement – i.e. my choice – alcohol was always involved.

On my last day's cycling, in Croatia, labouring my way up a steepish hill, I passed a primary school. A kid in the playground yelled at me, in Croatian, 'Hey fatty. Hurry up!' As a weight-loss measure, the whole thing had been a failure.

Six weeks after leaving Hamburg, I pedalled up to my aunt's block of flats in the eastern suburbs of Zagreb. I locked the bike up, unloaded my stuff, and sat in her little kitchen, drinking plum brandy and eating everything she put in front of me.

I had only started work experience at the BBC in March but, by December, Paul was brave enough to pack me off on a foreign trip, effectively to a war zone. Aware of my connection with the former Yugoslavia, he decided I should head off there to produce a series of films with a young reporter called David Willis. David went on to report from just about everywhere in the world, but this was his first overseas gig. Our initial stop was Belgrade. To get there we had to fly to Budapest and drive for six hours. After filming there for a couple of days, and eating and drinking together in the evening, I felt we had become firm friends.

Next came Zagreb where, as well as my aunt, I had many friends. I couldn't wait to bowl in there with my new BBC colleague and drink punishingly strong spirits half the night. We were only there for a day before catching an early flight to Dubrovnik the following morning. We met a few of my friends in the evening but David didn't want to drink. I recall feeling incredibly let down, concluding that we simply couldn't be the friends I thought we were; even that he wasn't the man I thought he was. All because he wasn't drinking. Absurd, simply absurd. Nearly thirty years later, even though he's worked out of California for most of that time, we're still in touch.

As for my friendship with Adam Shaw, the non-football fan with whom I presented *Working Lunch*, close as we were, and for all the time we spent together, I only ever felt we'd really cemented that friendship when I finally managed to get him to sit in a pub with me all afternoon. I knew he wasn't a big drinker, but every now and then he'd enjoy a heavy night out or a long lunch. This occasion was different. *Working Lunch* came off-air at 1pm. We had something to eat and then sat all afternoon in a pub called The Castle in Holland Park. We drank a huge amount, even for me. It was a memorable afternoon, which is an odd thing to say about an afternoon the specifics of which I have very little memory. It went on well into the evening, towards the end of which Adam got rather emotional talking about aspects of his life. I remember this so well because, to my shame really, I felt it was only at that moment that Adam and I truly bonded. I had subtly coerced him into drinking more than he wanted so he'd share with me more than he wanted. And now we were proper friends.

On the way home, I vomited in an upturned bin lid outside the Coronet cinema in Notting Hill. Why on earth that particular detail has stuck in my mind, I know not. As for Adam, unlike me he was working first thing the following morning. He recalls staggering around Notting Hill, out of cash, asking strangers for money for a cab home, explaining that he had to be up at the crack of dawn to present a business programme.

🍷 🥛 🥛

After eighteen months as a researcher in the business programmes department at Television Centre in West London, I went off to work on radio at Broadcasting House in central London. My first three months there were to be spent in the radio newsroom where the all-important news bulletins were produced. On my first day in this decidedly austere working environment, Brian Johnston, the great cricket commentator, passed away. I was entrusted with writing the newsreader's script to cue up a tribute that had been recorded with the cricketer Ian

Botham. This was for the prestigious thirty-minute 6pm news programme on Radio 4, which was referred to, reverently, as *the eighteen-hundred*. Crafting this intro was all I had to do all afternoon. They were happy because the new boy was being kept busy; I was happy because I was confident I could pull it off. A thirty-second script is less than a hundred words. Given my knowledge of cricket, all my journalistic training and the three hours I was given to discharge this task, I felt I had it in the bag. My work was duly passed up the chain of command for review and judged to be fit for broadcast.

At the pipping of the 6pm pips, I settled down at my desk to listen to my masterpiece go out. I'd called my parents, and everyone else I could think of, to tell them to do the same. The last words of my script, to get into the tape of Botham, were: 'Ian Botham added his voice to the chorus of tributes from the world of cricket.' Note the choice of words there, honed to perfection over three long hours. I was particularly pleased with 'chorus', a gentle nod perhaps towards a choir at the great man's funeral.

Unfortunately, the words 'the world of cricket' at the end of my intro were instantly replicated by Ian Botham, whose taped tribute began with the words 'The world of cricket has lost...' I winced. When the bulletin finished, the editor emerged from the studio and tapped me on the head with gentle severity. 'Double cue,' he said. 'Sounds ugly; don't let it happen again.' I reddened and stammered something halfway between an abject apology and a question along the lines of 'How come the dozen other people who checked it never saw it?'

He smiled and said, 'Come on, come for a drink.'

I shook my head and said I was working on the next major bulletin, at 10pm.

'So are we,' he said.

And, with that, three of his colleagues fell into step with him and off they went, repairing to the Yorkshire Grey just around the corner. Bewildered, I tailed after them; it literally seemed rude not to. As the newbie, with an ugly double cue to atone for to boot, I felt I should get the round in. This offer was waved away as they were in a round of their own. Plainly the four of them were in a four-pint arrangement and a fifth musketeer would confuse matters; if I joined the round that would necessitate the drinking of five pints instead of four, which I assumed they considered excessive. I suppose even four pints might be thought a bit on the high side for anyone charged with putting an important news bulletin out the same evening.

No, accomplished drinker as I was, this was too much for me. I enjoyed the pint they very kindly bought for me, promised them I'd not write another double cue that evening or ever again, and sloped off back to work to hold the fort while they put their four pints away. Before long they filed back into the newsroom to prepare the 22.00 bulletin, which passed without incident.

I tell this story to illustrate the kind of drinking culture that existed in my business in the last decade of the twentieth century. It's a story I've told often over the years to make this point but, recounting it now, I realise I had another purpose in doing so. It's one of the many stories I've told to support my claim that I wasn't a heavy or problem drinker. Me? A heavy drinker? You should have met these guys! All of us heavy drinkers like to have even heavier drinkers with whom we can compare ourselves. It makes us feel better about our own drinking.

🍷 🥛 🍺

I'm often asked what you need to do to become a presenter. My answer is always the same: find someone daft enough to give you something to present. That person for me was Alan Griffiths who was in charge of radio business programmes. To general bewilderment, he gave me some programmes to present on Radio 4 and the World Service. Before long, Radio 5 Live launched, and I got the gig presenting the early morning business news. This meant I was usually finished by mid-morning, which opened up all sorts of drinking possibilities.

As I had to be up for 3.30am, evenings out were tricky, so I drank all day instead. Over many long lunches I had many fascinating conversations with all sorts of brilliant people. There was the odd crashing bore, too, but the alcohol made them bearable. The intake of food and drink was ridiculous. At one lunch with a colleague at a French place in Knightsbridge, I ate a phenomenal amount of goose pâté washed down with a lot of wine. I then met another friend in a pub late in the afternoon and stayed there until about 9pm before staggering home and collapsing fully clothed into bed. I woke up feeling like a great greasy ball of goose fat and toxins but still managed to roll into work before 4am. I daresay I came off-air, had a big breakfast and was back with my head in a glass by lunchtime.

Occasionally, a few like-minded souls hatched plans for more ambitious post-breakfast-show boozing. Someone heard tell of pubs around Smithfield Market, licensed to open at breakfast time to slake the thirst of butchers coming off the early shift. This was before strict rules on opening times were dropped, so the prospect greatly excited us. We'd sometimes repair there after our early shifts and join the meat men downing pints of lager and getting stuck into bacon sandwiches. It was paradise. I'd usually get home at lunchtime and sleep the sleep of the dead for a few hours. On occasion, the breakfast session turned into a lunchtime session and afternoon session and even on into the evening. Somehow, I'd still be up with the sparrows for work at around 3.30 the following morning.

These glorious morning sessions had to become a thing of the past when my old boss on TV, Paul Gibbs, launched a lunchtime business programme called *Working Lunch*. To the consternation/alarm of everyone, he chose me to present it. So after the 4am start for the early shift on 5 Live, I'd then have to clock in at 9am to prepare for *Working Lunch*, which went out live at 12.30.

There's a tape of the first show somewhere. Though I was well into my twenties, I look as though I might not be old enough to do a paper round. I flap my arms about randomly as I talk to camera, possibly in a subconscious effort to ventilate my armpits which are ringed with huge patches of sweat. By the end of the show I'm pretty much soaked through.

Somehow we survived the first few weeks and months of this occasionally madcap production. The technology we used to create a kind of virtual studio was all new and often crashed. It was terrifying and thrilling in equal measure.

This seemed to communicate itself to the guests, some of whom were less comfortable in this chaotic environment than others. One contributor took a funny turn just before I was supposed to be interviewing him live. A producer sprinted upstairs from the studio into Paul's office where he was in a meeting with some high-up or other. She went straight for the bottom drawer of his desk where she knew he kept some emergency whisky, whipped the bottle out, and ran back to the studio. The medicine was administered, and the poor chap was broadcasting to the nation with me a few minutes later. Quite how Paul's meeting progressed, I cannot recall.

It wasn't just the odd contributor in need of alcohol. On more days than not, the programme was followed by drinking. Sometimes just one or two in the office, often a lot more than that. There was a wine bar a short walk down Wood Lane called Albertines. Over the years the wine consumed by BBC people in that place would have filled Lake Windermere. Tales were told of legendary boozers, many famous names among them, drinking Olympian quantities day and night, falling asleep under a table, going straight to work in the morning and then doing it all over again. Impressive, or quite mad. Either way, as ever, it was nice to have knowledge of drinkers whose intake cast my own in a favourable light.

Another regular haunt for a while was a place we called 'The Turkish', on the Goldhawk Road. It was a glorified kebab shop which sold plates of meat, cold beer and cheap wine. I had many a long lunch in there with television journalists I liked and admired. I'd never known happiness like it. I was in my late twenties, enjoying undreamed of success in a business I never dared to imagine getting into, and wildly, happily drunk on a weekday afternoon. Sheer bliss.

One afternoon, after a brilliant couple of hours in there with Paul Gibbs, talking about work, family, life and everything, we fell into silence watching people walk past going about whatever their business was. Paul said, 'Do you ever look at the rest of the world and wonder exactly what they do?'

I nodded and said I did. What I was thinking was how miserable it must be to be in a job in which you can't drink all afternoon and have conversations like this.

The place we went to most often was a pub-restaurant in Holland Park called The Academy. It was run by a Croatian guy I knew called Darko. The afternoon hours we spent in there don't bear thinking about. On the evening of my thirtieth birthday I had a party there. I arrived for this function unfashionably early, straight after the show at 1.30. A few of us settled in for the afternoon and carried right on until more of our colleagues showed up in the evening. A quite famous presenter had already been drinking elsewhere when he turned up. He ordered a meal, ate it, and shortly afterwards vomited in the street outside.

Thereafter he was right as rain. He carried on drinking for a couple of hours more before getting peckish again and ordering another meal. This one he kept down. Impressive.

Again it was nice to be with someone who was worse than... etc. You get the point.

Twenties drinks scorecard

● POSSIBLE INTERVENTIONS

Two things could have changed my path. Perhaps as a result of some health issue, a doctor could have taken me aside and gently told me I was drinking too much and why it would be worth cutting down a bit. They might have added that I could enjoy a drink, and really go for it on occasions, but if I wanted to continue to do so long term, I'd need to find a way of drinking less in total.

● CONSUMPTION

Massive. For this and my next two decades there weren't many days I didn't drink something. So, as a baseline, I was drinking the equivalent of two pints of beer a day, 35 units a week, just for starters. Those big sessions would involve, on top of that, at least a bottle of wine, and around, I'd say, three more pints. So that, being generous with myself here, is 10 units for the wine and about 8 for the beer. 18 units. I would say there were two or three of these sessions a week. I'll call it an average of two and a half sessions a week. 18 multiplied by 2.5 gives us 45 units. So that's 35 'base' units and 45 'session' units. All up: **80 units a week**. Blimey.

● BORING BITS

Not many I can recall. Sometimes I'd only continue drinking because I was too knackered to do anything else. Slumped in the back of cabs night after night, trying to keep traffic lights from appearing in double vision, I reflected that things were getting a bit samey as well as a little out of hand. There were parties and work functions where I drank through the boredom, but generally everything seemed to stay new and thrilling right through my twenties.

● PROPORTION OF DRINKS WANTED/NEEDED/ENJOYED
80 per cent.

His name is John and he is a moderator

John Robins, late thirties, is a comedian, alcohol lover, pub enthusiast. He could hardly be more different to Llana, our previous moderator, in his approach. While she has become indifferent to alcohol, his love for it is undiminished. To get to where he is now, he's spent a of lot of time thinking about why he drinks, what he drinks and how he drinks. I like what he says in answer to the first of those three questions:

> *It connects you to so many times of your life. Even when you're in your living room having a bottle of wine on your own, there's a sort of a sense memory of like being out with your friends, or something you did at school, or a mate you drank with or something, It's really interesting; it's like nostalgia.*

These are feelings I'm familiar with. In his time, in short, he's drunk loads, stopped, gone back to drinking loads again, stopped again, started drinking loads again, and then finally sorted himself out. While really enthusiastic boozers may have read Llana's story without much relish, John's tells a different tale. There's more than one way to skin the cat of moderation.

Before I went to uni my problem was gambling. As a teenager I did twelve steps recovery and so on for that, but not for booze. I don't remember drinking becoming like a daily thing until I was at uni. And then when I came back from uni, I was working in a bookshop and I started drinking very heavily, to excess every night. I never thought about it in terms of units, obviously, but I was probably at around 80 or 90 units a week.

It was basically when I did my first ever stand-up gig that I realised I had to quit drinking, so I stopped. Apart from anything else I needed to drive to gigs and stuff. It's quite weird to think now, that there were periods when I was abstinent. But the amount of comedy gigs that allowed me to do when I first started out was amazing. I mean, that was the hardest I've ever worked at my job.

Yet he went back to drinking, and heavily, before stopping again for eight months. But soon the lure of the pub proved too much and off he went once more.

While I was abstinent I'd basically had to stop going to pubs because I realised very quickly there was no point in being sober in a pub for more than half an hour, an hour. I just didn't feel part of it. The fact is, I love pubs. I adore everything about them: the history, the community traditions, the literature about drinking. So, I started again in 2012. Then at Christmas 2016 my girlfriend left me. I was alone in the house and basically I had a real moment when I thought, you need to stop, you need to do Dry January, or this is going to be an absolute car crash. And I did it, I did Dry January and I was really proud that I was able to do that.

And when I started drinking again at the start of February, I said to myself, OK, if you're going to drink now, you're going to have to manage it. So I immediately stopped drinking spirits and banned them from the house. That was my killer – rum and coke. That was a really important step in managing my drinking, realising that when I poured myself a pint of rum and coke it had four shots in it. And I was having three of those every evening. Essentially, I was drinking 12 units a night even before I counted any beer and wine I drank. I also opt for the weakest beer in a pub when I'm out, and never have anything above 4.5 per cent abv in the house, usually ale somewhere between 3 and 4 per cent.

The issue with excessive drinking is that those in the grip of it are generally considered to be incapable of rational thought about it. John's experience suggests otherwise, and we haven't got on to the clever bit yet. It's not a technique I'd heard of before, though I have come across it since.

I had this silly calendar, from the writers' room of The Last Leg. It was like a joke one with pictures on it of all the people who worked on the show. I'd got myself a red Sharpie and marked off every day as I got through January. It helped me because it did kind of highlight what I was achieving. I thought that since I'd often beaten myself up about how much I drink, it was important to actually celebrate when I managed not to. And that sort of aide memoire got me through January. And then I just thought, you know what, I'm going to carry this on throughout the year, marking up all the days I don't drink. I made up my mind to not drink on at

*least another 100 days that year. In the end, in total, I didn't
drink for 137 days that year, and I've bettered that since.*

This idea has the merit of being prescriptive, yet flexible.
John can see how many non-drinking days he has left to
mark up before the end of the year and adjust his drinking
accordingly. To clock up the magic 100 days before New Year's
Eve he has to put in an average of eight or nine dry days a
month. If he's not hitting that, he'll be facing the possibility
of having to carve out a lot of drink-free days in December,
so that's one incentive to get them in the bag earlier. I've done
something similar in the past: doing a deal with myself that
if I had a drinking day, I'd then have the next day off. If I had
two drinking days, then I'd make sure I had two days off. This
can work because, again, it's flexible. Let's say I was on holiday
for a week and drank too much every day, then I would have
a whole week off it and even things up again. Importantly, it
should also mean that you're getting the benefit of more than
180 drink-free days a year.

The danger with this approach is the temptation to not
'waste' a drinking day on one or two sensible drinks. I've certainly been guilty of thinking along the lines of, well, today's a
drinking day, so I might as well make the most of it and really
get tanked up. In which case you're somewhat missing the point
of the exercise. Still, I think it's worth a try.

The other issue here, which will have many a therapist
tutting away, is that neither John nor I are, as they might see
it, addressing the root causes of our drinking, whatever they
might be. And without doing so all these strategies will prove
worthless in the end. I take the point, I suppose, as we both
plainly still have alcohol too high up on that pedestal. But,
again, whatever works, works. Even if the whole process is
exhausting; his hundred or more dry days a year are hard-won.

I definitely find it harder having the first night off after I've been drinking. And sometimes, kind of, I feel a bit pathetic because I really have to sort of almost talk myself through it. I was in the supermarket the other day and I was agonising over whether I should have that night off. Because when you start to keep track of your drinking days, the non-drinking days really kind of stand out. I need to start talking myself into it, saying, I've got to be up early, or there's no reason for me to drink tonight because I'm on my own. Or I'm drinking this weekend so this is one of the nights I must have off.

Then I'm walking around the supermarket, and I see a guy with, you know, four Stellas, or a woman with a bottle of wine and I start thinking, well, they're doing it, why shouldn't I? But that's a stupid way of looking at it; it could be his only drink of the week, or she might well have bought it to take to a dinner party. She's not necessarily going home to get smashed on her own.

Some people think it is a bit weird that I go to all these lengths. I had a girlfriend who didn't drink and I think she found it difficult when I was distracted about whether I could drink or not. She didn't have a problem with me having a drink, but she did notice how much time I spent focusing on not doing it. When I was trying to have a night off I could be anxious, especially around new people, or preoccupied. The nights I wasn't drinking were probably more difficult than the nights when I was. Though she always said she'd never actually seen me drunk. I guess that's the tolerance, which isn't a good sign.

This is a new one on me. I've heard it said several times that if you're thinking about not drinking all the time, that is extremely unsatisfactory and a clear sign that you're not in control. John dares to turn that on its head, in effect saying, 'Yes, drinking preoccupies me whether I'm drinking or not, and I like it like that.' Sub-optimal? Yes, but does this way of looking at it help him moderate his intake? Yes again, so what of it?

Two other 'policies' of John's gave me pause for thought:

A big thing for me is trying not to have the last drink of the night, because the last drink of the night is only getting you drunk when you're in bed. So it's probably making your hangover worse while you're not actually getting any of the benefit, if you can call it a benefit. Either way, it's a pointless drink because you won't get to experience any of the alcohol.

I'd never thought of that. He's right, and I salute the fact that he is apparently capable of such rational thought so late in the evening. I will endeavour to do the same. John told me that when he watched my drinking documentary it was like watching a film about himself. And the similarities do mount up.

In terms of my drinking pattern I never drink in the day.

Nor me now.

I never drink at lunchtime.

And again.

And I'm never in a pub garden at two in the afternoon because I just don't like it; it makes me feel tired.

Well, I couldn't say 'never' with my hand on my heart, but only rarely, and it definitely puts me out of action for the rest of the day.

But what I do get, around four o'clock or five o'clock, is a real kind of thirst on.

165

Yes, yes and yes again. At that time of day, for me too, the desire to be in a pub with a pint of beer in my hand becomes overwhelming. If I can get to around seven o'clock without giving in to the urge, I'm generally fine. I suppose that must mean that for me, as for John, it's more about the pubs than the beer. I'm lucky in that, once I get past the early evening hump, I'm not tempted to reach into the fridge at home; the moment has passed. John has his own way of getting past his early evening hump.

Once I've eaten, it kind of breaks the spell. So, I try to eat a big meal at around five, and the rest of the evening I find so much easier.

This caused me to take a long hard look at myself. I always eat later than is good for me, and it shocks me to realise why: I've never much fancied a drink, especially beer, once I've eaten. So, over many years, I believe I've gradually got into the habit of eating late for fear of spoiling the drinking.

I've tried to address this recently and found it really hard to change my ways. Even if I'm not planning on going out drinking, I still can't seem to bring myself to eat earlier. I find this rather shaming. Not least because the easiest route for me to get over my early evening drinking humps was staring me in the face. It's just that I was too blinded by the light shining down on me from the pint of beer up on that pedestal.

There are many therapists who would look at John (and me) and conclude that we are kidding ourselves if we think we have conquered whatever alcohol dependency issues we have. They may be right, but if this way of living alongside – rather than conquering – his appetite for alcohol works for John, that's good enough for me. I salute his efforts.

I know I'm still drinking an unhealthy amount, so I do need to try for more days off. But something I think I also need to address is making sure that on nights when I'm not drinking, I'm as attentive, bubbly and talkative as I am when I'm having a drink.

Quite right too. And it's plainly an important commitment to make. I suppose it also raises the question that if it's possible to be just as attentive, bubbly and talkative without taking a drink, then why take the drink in the first place? That's a question for me as well as for John, and I don't really have an answer. I suspect we've spent so long believing that it's alcohol helping us to be the fun, interesting kind of guys we hope we are that we can't quite shake that conviction – even when we're presented with evidence that it is possible for us to be charming enough company without it.

🍷 🥛 🍺

Postscript: Moderator no more

After the first edition of this book came out, John Robins got in touch with me and asked if he could add a postscript to this chapter. Here's what he wants to say:

What you've just read is based on an interview with Adrian in the summer of 2020. At that point I had been attempting to seriously moderate my drinking for nearly four years. I was delighted to discuss my strategies as it had become something of an obsession of mine. However, since then I have come to realise that though this obsession was reducing my alcohol intake, it had begun to dominate most of my waking hours. I was thinking about alcohol all the time, and this was having a serious impact on my mental health, work and relationships.

Towards the end of 2021 most of the strategies we discussed went out of the window and I was back to the daily drinking I had tried so hard to avoid. Something had to be done. As I write this now, I am one hundred and fourteen days sober, and have come to understand that my obsession with moderating my alcohol intake, far from providing evidence that I was in control of my drinking, proved that I wasn't.

The following passage had a huge impact on me, and changed the way I viewed my attempts at moderation: 'The idea that somehow, someday he will control and enjoy his drinking is the great obsession of every abnormal drinker. The persistence of this illusion is astonishing. Many pursue it into the gates of insanity or death.' (Alcoholics Anonymous p.30)

I think about these words every day. It's not that I think all attempts at moderation are futile, far from it. I wouldn't dream of dissuading anyone from taking time to consider a lot of what we covered in this chapter. Moderation may well be your path to a more healthy relationship with alcohol and a happier life.

In my case, though moderation was possible for a time, it did not address the mental and spiritual damage alcohol was causing me. If anything, it intensified it. That said, I do so hope you are able to control and enjoy your drinking. In the end I found I could do neither.

John Robins, March 2023

For the love of drinking, drink less

If I'd known I was going to live this long I'd have looked after myself better.

Tommy Docherty, footballer and manager, 1928–2020

Drinking has been the focus of my social life since my mid-teens. If a night out didn't involve alcohol, I wouldn't much fancy it. I'd probably give it a miss completely. And I'm afraid that remained as true at the age of fifty as it was at fifteen. I've had many great times along the way, but I do harbour this regret: I'm sure I could have had just as great a time while drinking an awful lot less.

As I've said, all the drinks I've put away in my life, laid out in a line, would stretch about three miles. But how many of all those drinks did I really enjoy, want or need?

Psychologists say you should never really need a drink, as such. But there's something worse than needing a drink: that's drinking a drink you don't need or want or enjoy. If I walk along my three-mile line of drinks I'm appalled to realise that by the one-mile mark I'm already seeing drinks I could have managed without; drinks I could have not drunk without diminishing my enjoyment of anything one jot.

Let's put a figure on my proportion of 'essential' drinking. I've got it at 30 per cent. So, 70 per cent of what I've glugged has been for nothing. Two miles of drinks for nothing. What an idiot. And not only have I gained nothing by squirting that lot through my system, I have to consider the downsides: the money, the calories and the detrimental effect on my physical and mental health.

To punish myself for my stupidity I have considered abstinence, but there's too much about drinking that I enjoy. So I resolved to find a way of living my drinking life in the beautiful 30 per cent of the drinks I want and leaving the pointless 70 per cent behind. I always want to be able to take a quiet early evening pint or two with a friend; share a bottle of wine over dinner somewhere, and, yes, occasionally drink too much at a wedding, say something inappropriate to a relative of the bride, and dance with wild incompetence.

This is the greatest motivation I have for cutting down, because I never want to get to the stage where doctors are telling me I mustn't touch another drop. If and when I get into shuffling old age, I want to be able to stagger to a pub and drink a pint or two. I want to be able to sit alone there reading something. Or just sit there, staring watery-eyed into space. Or I could shoot the breeze with one of my old codger mates. Or dispense worldly wisdom to some unfortunate youth I've collared who's too polite to walk away. Yes, I could do all this without a pint in my hand, but I'd much prefer for it not to have to be that way.

Paul Cook, drummer with the Sex Pistols, happens to drink in one of my locals. After my TV documentary about drinking went out, he often asked me about his intake.

'I just enjoy a couple of pints,' he'd say sheepishly, as though he was checking to see if that was OK with me. I told him I thought that after what he'd been through in the seventies, a couple of pints most nights was small potatoes. I asked him how come he'd never been addicted to heroin back in the day.

'I was,' he said.

'How did you get off it?'

He shrugged. 'Dunno, just did.'

'The tragedy of heroin,' he said, 'is that it's wasted on young idiots like I was. When you need it is when you're old and knackered and your leg's hurting and stuff. I'll be on the gear all day long when I'm like that.'

I doubt he was being entirely serious, but I'm deadly serious that I'll make sure to keep in touch with him just in case. It's this idea I'm channelling with drink. In the twilight of my life, when I really want it, need it and will most definitely enjoy it, I would like to be able to have it.

🍷🥛🍺

Just as everyone's got a different idea of what constitutes moderate drinking, there's plenty of disagreement as to what heavy drinking looks like. My own view is as follows. Based on no scientific expertise but plenty of reading, and discussions with countless medics and drinkers (and some drinking medics), if you're dropping much more than 35 units a week – around fifteen drinks – you're a heavy drinker.

And the longer you go on as a heavy drinker, the greater the risk that, sooner or later, someone's going to raise a sign reading, 'STOP, OR ELSE'. Rolling along at north of twice that intake, I reckon I was firmly in this category. In five or ten years, the way I was going, it was clear to me that I'd have had to stop completely or face some pretty dire consequences with my innards.

I didn't want to get to that stage, and neither did I want to get to the stage where I was quite unable to find a way of drinking less. After all, I think it's reasonable to assume that the longer you go on drinking heavily, the harder it will be to cut down in the end.

I went through a phase of marathon running in my thirties. It was more staggering than running, to be fair, but I got myself around four marathons. One of the many benefits was that it was yet another stupid excuse not to curtail my drinking – 'See, I do all this running, so I'm sweating all the booze out anyway.' But I remember reading somewhere how important it was to stay hydrated. One line particularly stuck with me: 'If you're feeling thirsty, it's almost too late: your body is already dehydrated. Your thirst is your body's way of telling you that, so take on water even if you don't feel you need it yet.'

In a similar vein, I once interviewed a counsellor with Relate, the marriage guidance charity. She said that the hardest thing in her business was that by the time couples came to her for her help, it was already too late; the damage had been done and so it was that much harder to repair. Ever since I had that conversation, I've been tempted to buy a course of ten sessions with Relate for all newlyweds of my acquaintance. I reckon one every six months for the first five years of marriage should be enough to stop any rot setting in. Needless to say, I've never had the guts to go through with this idea.

All of which is my long-winded way of saying that if you're a heavy drinker, even if you're experiencing (as I did) no noticeable ill effects, think about moderating while you can. Because there's a fair chance that one day, if you don't, moderation won't be an option. It will all be too late; you'll just have to do without.

For the love of drinking itself, it's worth considering.

Thirties

On my thirtieth birthday, a dear friend of mine, a man then in his sixties, tapped me gently on the shoulder and said, 'Just so you know, thirty to forty goes by in the blink of an eye.' He was right. And forty to fifty goes even more quickly (we'll come to that). I don't know if those years were sped up by all the drinking I was doing, but it certainly swallowed up a lot of time.

Apart from anything else, there seemed to be a wedding to go to at least once a month. And for every wedding there was the mandatory stag weekend, when of course there was mandatory drinking to be done. I viewed these events with the same disdain I have for New Years' Eve. They were for amateur drinkers to go berserk; this kind of rumbustious special occasion drinking was for dilettantes.

Most of these stags involved people drawn from the same circle of friends. Possibly as a means of differentiating each one of these events from the next, they got progressively more extreme. Oddly enough, I was generally the sensible one. It was me who freed a naked Kev after he'd been taped to a traffic light in Edinburgh. And it was me who literally kidnapped my brother from his own stag in Tintagel, so worried was I for his welfare. On each occasion I incurred the wrath of the rest of the group for being a spoilsport.

On the one hand I stand by my common-sense actions; on the other I can see that this might have been my way of kidding myself and others that I was the good, responsible, adult drinker and everyone should take note of it.

My stag, incidentally, for reasons unclear, took place in Swindon. I was dressed up in a Batman outfit made of wool, to which I'm allergic. I spent a long weekend damp from the beer I was soaked in, and itching like mad. I've not been back to Swindon since.

🍷🥃🍺

In my thirties I got married and had two daughters and was presenting television and radio programmes six days a week. It was a busy time. There are 3,652 days in a decade and throughout this one I doubt there were more than a hundred during which I didn't have a drink. Usually not much, frequently a fair amount, sometimes an awful lot. It never seemed to be a problem. I always got to work, and work was going really well. I was doing a fair amount of drinking in the afternoon but, as my working day finished at 1pm, that didn't seem especially unreasonable. Nobody would have thought I had a problem, least of all the people I was drinking with.

Inconveniently, the more successful I got, the more unhappy I seemed to get. I suppose I put this down to the pressure of work, the mind-bending business of fame, and the slow collapse of my marriage. All of these were obviously linked, but I never considered alcohol to be part of the story. If I gave my intake any thought at all I would have seen it as just part of my life, and not something I could do without at this exciting but difficult time.

When the girls were little, their mum, Jane, presented her radio show in the afternoon, so we had a babysitter in to look after them until I got back some time after *Working Lunch* came off-air at one o'clock. Often, but not often enough, I was home by mid-afternoon, sent the nanny on her way, and did the playing, feeding and bathing myself. I wish I'd done more of this.

With more work suddenly coming my way, I was often out filming something. I also played an indecent amount of golf and did a lot of running. I never felt I needed an excuse to drink in the evenings, but if I'd been working, golfing or running all afternoon I'd definitely feel as if I'd earned it. If I'd been parenting all afternoon I'd feel as if I'd earned it too. And if I'd been drinking all afternoon, I doubtless thought I might just as well crack on into the evening.

Sometimes, after they'd had their tea, I'd take the girls, in a sling or a pram or whatever, out for a walk. We'd usually end up in my local. I'd take a pint or two while young Polish barmaids and old barflies alike cooed at my offspring.

Long lunches were occasionally organised by the hard drinkers of the BBC's sports department. One of my most entertaining colleagues of that era was a brilliant Irish lad called Fergus Sweeney. As one of these sports lunches lurched from the afternoon into the evening, Fergus and I got involved in an Irish Coffee drinking competition. I seem to recall that it finished with a 14-14 score draw. I was in bed at midnight but at four in the morning I was still wide awake, sweating, with a headache, and my heart beating out of my chest.

The first football World Cup I covered was Germany 2006. Gary Lineker was the main presenter. I was a very distant number two – Baldrick to his Blackadder. This bothered me not a jot because I had an absolute ball. Every other day, I presented the highlights programme. Other than that, I drank and drank and drank. If not at lunchtime, then certainly in the evening, unless I was working in the evening, in which case I'd join my colleagues in whatever bar they were in after the show finished. Either way, the drinking would go on long into the night.

Then I'd get up in the morning and do it all over again. I was away for a month, during which time I can't imagine I put away less than 500 units of alcohol. However late I got in, I'd set the alarm so I could ring home and catch the girls before they went to school. This was also designed to convey that, as I was awake at a reasonable hour, I can't have been up half the night. But one morning I made the call, opened my mouth to talk and, as it was so dry, nothing came out. I had to cough and retch to clear my throat. I fear this gave me away. On all subsequent mornings, to ensure my voice was functioning, I'd spend a few moments doing some vocal exercises before making the call.

I don't think I disgraced myself during this orgy of drinking. The only time I came close was with Mick McCarthy, the Irish ex-international player and manager, and his wife Fiona, both of whom I liked very much. I'd been out drinking for heaven knows how long and had rounded the night off with a classic German-Turkish kebab. When I rolled into the hotel bar, gone midnight, Mick, who was working with the BBC, introduced me to Fiona, who'd just arrived in Berlin. I kissed her on both cheeks – and was horrified to see my lips had left significant grease upon them. Before either she, Mick or I knew what I was doing, I'd whipped out a handkerchief and was wiping her face.

As drunken exploits go, this wasn't like waking up in a bed with three strangers, but I still shudder at the thought. I'm sure Fiona does too.

I also have a physical injury to serve as a reminder of this time. Late one night as I was trotting up some stone steps towards the door of a casino, I tripped, fell and smashed my left elbow very hard indeed. It bled copiously, which was reason enough for the doorman to deny my entrance to the casino. To this day, when I lean on this elbow a searing pain like an electric shock can rear up my arm, causing me to yelp in distress. Serves me right, or *dient mir richtig* as they say in Germany.

Throughout my fourth decade I know I drank almost every day because the non-drinking days were so rare that they've stuck fast in my mind. There was the week I didn't drink before running the London Marathon, for example, which felt like as big a challenge as the race itself. Then there was the Lent I abstained from alcohol. This felt like a really massive achievement too. The first drink I had was a whisky at just before midnight on Easter Saturday. I remember it vividly even though it was nearly twenty years ago. That's how big a deal it was.

Something else I recall vividly is an appointment with my GP. I can't remember what it was for, but something made me ponder on how I'd react if he told me I had to stop drinking. I remember very clearly concluding that this would be nothing short of an absolute disaster for me. An absolute disaster.

As it turned out, he said nothing of the sort, but I retrospectively diagnose myself as seriously dependent on alcohol. I wish he had said something, although obviously he couldn't have done so, given that I wouldn't have told him how much I was putting away.

Thirties drinks scorecard

● POSSIBLE INTERVENTIONS

Short of some real drink-related health crisis, I can't think of anything that would have worked. A life without alcohol was by now so unthinkable that I can even remember the moment I realised it was unthinkable.

● CONSUMPTION

Huge. I would be downing a minimum of a pint of beer and the best part of a bottle of wine every day. My then wife didn't drink much, so if the bottle was finished, which it usually was, I'd have drunk most of it. That's 2.5 units for the beer, minimum, and at least 6 units worth of wine. 8.5 multiplied by 7 days is 59.5 which we'll round up to 60. Add to this a long lunch or two and at least a couple of heavy nights out and we're looking at north of **100 units a week**.

● BORING BITS

The drinking around work, especially the football, was invariably great. And though I loved my local, I was aware of it getting a bit samey, having similar conversations with the same people night in night out. At home, eating and drinking for hours on end got boring in itself. I was eating to drink and drinking to eat. After each evening meal I'd pile in cheese and biscuits and wine and more cheese and more biscuits and more wine before eventually wobbling up to bed.

● PROPORTION OF DRINKS WANTED/NEEDED/ENJOYED

70 per cent.

Beige

Sometimes a single sentence or just a solitary word can change your way of thinking.

I've got a friend who, like nearly all my friends, likes a drink. She doesn't have a particularly happy relationship with alcohol.

'I've made many terrible decisions in my life, and alcohol has always been part of them,' is one thing she says.

Another is, 'If I only had five pounds left, I would spend it on wine, rather than buy myself some food.'

As ever, I took this as more reassuring evidence that my drinking wasn't as bad as somebody else's.

She said something else that really appalled me, something which marked a turning point in my drinking life. I was on the phone to her sometime after a Lent during which I'd not touched alcohol. I was telling her what I had enjoyed about it: the freedom from the temptations of all the drinking options normally open to me, and all the time that had become available to spend doing other things. I also told her what I'd missed: the craic on a big night, the quiet pint here and there, and so on. In general, I explained, it had been a really positive experience, and I'd cut down a lot when I started drinking again but, by now, I was back to drinking as much as I'd ever drunk.

'The problem,' she said. 'Is that when I don't drink, the world seems a very beige place to me.'

Beige? I thought this was an awful thing to say and, even worse, I realised that I felt the same way. How could we have drunk our way into a state of mind in which alcohol had convinced us that the world was colourless without it?

I was sitting on a bench in the park opposite my flat as we had this conversation. I looked up, down and around. Beige? The sky was so blue and the trees so green that they almost hurt to behold. The vivid beauty of the colours felt like a reproach. I pictured all my family and friends, with all the fun, beauty, love and wisdom they brought to me, and saw that they weren't beige either. Yet I would have looked forward to seeing each and every one of them a little bit more if there was drink involved. I felt nothing less than ashamed. Something had to change.

At some point, most drinkers ask themselves if they have a problem. Are they dependent on alcohol? How much is too much? Are they 'alcoholics'? There are many criteria, none conclusive in my opinion. If you drink all day every day then, yes, you probably have serious issues. And the same is true if you show physical signs of withdrawal – the shakes and so on – if you don't drink. But there are other indicators too; for example if you, like me, have convinced yourself it takes a drink inside you to put colour into your world.

What I wish more doctors would say

What's the definition of an alcoholic?
Someone who drinks more than their doctor.

TIRED OLD JOKE. ANON.

I had a good GP at one time whom I liked and respected very much. She was really kind to me at a difficult time in my life. I liked her way with words. Once, when she prescribed me some new long-term medication for something or other, I bemoaned the fact that I was taking no fewer than four different pills. 'Welcome to middle age,' she said. (I'm now on six daily pills, by the way, so I'm much deeper into middle age.) As with more or less every other doctor I've spoken to, we worked with the usual tissue of lies regarding how much I drank: I probably said I drank between 20 and 30 units a week; she probably wrote down 40 to 50 units a week, and the truth was probably closer to 60 or 70 units a week. This much was understood.

I've had similar conversations with various specialists. There was the psychologist I saw to address my issues with anxiety and depression; the gastroenterologist who thrust a tube down my throat to determine why I often had a sensation of battery acid bubbling up inside my torso; and there was the cardiologist I went to about my blood pressure. In each case, even though alcohol is an important factor in all three areas – psychological matters, reflux and hypertension – they never got to the bottom of my drinking. While I lay the blame for this firmly at my own door, I can't help wishing these doctors had been more determined to kick that door down.

At my GP's one morning, to her dismay I'm sure, I presented with haemorrhoids. Unpleasant as they are, I never much mind getting them as it gives me the chance to boast to a medical professional that in *Viz* magazine my name is rhyming slang for piles. A lad is pictured grasping his bottom, wailing that his Adrians are giving him hell. That bit of fun out of the way, and having had a gentle prod around my fundament, she asked me if I strained much when I was on the toilet.

'No more than anyone else, I think,' is what I said, although how could I have known?

A few moments later she'd pulled her gloves off, I'd pulled my trousers up and she was giving me her verdict.

'I think you probably are straining,' she said. 'And I expect that's because you're dehydrated the morning after you've had a drink the night before.'

I nodded gravely, as she added: 'If you're really on it, then make sure you drink a lot of water too.'

On it? While I welcomed the use of the vernacular here, I can't imagine it was the kind of language doctors are taught to use at medical school. I remember hearing an exchange between an ex-footballer and his co-presenter at the conclusion of their morning radio show. He was asked what he was doing for the rest of the day.

'Oh, I'm on it,' he said, before outlining his plans, which, as I remember, involved going straight out on the lash well before lunchtime, and staying 'on it' for a good deal of the afternoon. Again, while I loved this shameless, devil-may-care relish at the prospect of a day lost to drink, I could recognise its dangers.

And here I was hearing my GP talk about being 'on it' too, and the importance of drinking plenty of water on those occasions. This was, obviously, sensible advice issued in a language I could understand, but putting it like this had unintended consequences. For a start, it kind of implied that the ingestion of water would somehow dilute the toxicity of the alcohol, which plainly isn't the case. The important point is that when she used the expression 'on it', she to some extent legitimised the act of being 'on it'. And we all know what 'on it' means: a proper session. I'm afraid that at some level, next time I was 'on it', I probably said to myself, 'Great, I'm now "on it", and my doctor knows about it, so it can't be terrible, but I must remember to drink plenty of water.'

Again, mea culpa, no question. But here's how I wish she'd put it:

'Mr Chiles, you have piles.' And we'd have a little laugh at this, before she'd continue thus:

It's not the worst case I've ever seen but you do need to be careful. I think you're probably straining a lot on the toilet. If your diet's good, which I know it is, it might be that, if and when you drink too much alcohol, it's leaving you dehydrated. I know that you, like me to be honest, drink a bit too much – a lot too much on occasion – and I'm sure you realise that sooner or later this will cause you problems, if it isn't already. After all, I see you're already on medication for depression, reflux and hypertension. No-one can say for sure that alcohol's causing those problems, but it definitely won't be helping. So please do try to cut down a bit – even just five pints less a week will be of massive benefit to you. But, let's be honest, you're still going to have the odd big night out. When you do, make sure you drink plenty of water, so you don't get dehydrated and constipated. But really, do try to cut down a good bit, because otherwise, in the end, piles could well be the least of your problems.

I think that would have been better.

🍷 🥃 🍺

I am generally in awe of doctors, and this particular GP was really great with me in all sorts of areas I needn't mention now, but here are some things I might humbly suggest that doctors, especially GPs, consider saying to drinkers like me:

- *I'll be honest with you, I drink too much as well, so I'm kind of talking to myself here as much as to you.*

- *Please be honest with me about how much you drink. I need you to really work it out for me. A very small glass of wine, a shot of spirits or half a pint of not-very-strong beer are all about one unit. So, nip back to the waiting room while I see my next patient and really try to work it out for me. Please be honest with me and yourself and then we can work out where to go from there. Don't panic! I'm not going to tell you to stop completely, or that you're going to drop dead anytime soon. I just want to help you. You might even end up enjoying drinking more.*

- *The trouble is, we've all got this idea of what an 'alcoholic' looks like – falling down drunk; drinking sherry in the morning etc. etc., but that really is misleading. In fact, we're trying to get away from the idea of 'the alcoholic' altogether because it confuses matters. Most of us who drink way too much end up comparing ourselves favourably to the image of the man in the shop doorway. And we decide that, as we're not like that, we're probably fine. Which quite possibly isn't true. I would class someone who is dangerously addicted to alcohol as a drinker who gets some kind of physical reaction – the shakes or whatever – when they don't drink. That's only ever going to be a tiny number of people, and I don't think you're one of them. But that doesn't mean you don't drink too much or that you're not to some extent dependent on it.*

- *The safe level of drinking is 14 units a week, which is a bottle and a half of wine or around seven pints of beer. Believe it or not, most drinkers do drink as little as that. I suspect you, like me, think 14 units is impossible to get to. Well, whatever, but let's set that aside. You're currently drinking more than 50 units a week. If you can just get it down to 30 you'll be doing your health an enormous favour. Please don't throw your hands in the air and give up just because you think you can't get it down to 14.*

- *Our age group – the middle-aged, essentially – are now the biggest drinkers. And we take a bigger risk with our drinking than younger drinkers. It's younger drinkers who tend to get all the attention, because they're usually noisy, anti-social and generally objectionable. But in terms of the adverse effect alcohol has on them, their youth is an advantage. If you're twenty and doing a lot of boozing, it probably won't be doing you a lot of good and it will be increasing your risk of things like liver disease and cancer. However, at that age, those risks will be low in the first place. Middle-aged drinkers like us are a different kettle of fish; because of our age, our chances of getting the bad stuff are already higher before we even touch a drop of alcohol. Throw in some proper drinking and you take your risk levels to somewhere you don't want them to be. You're probably not dicing with death exactly, but it's worth thinking about.*

Obviously, you enjoy a drink. And I take it that you'll always want to be able to enjoy a drink. The risk is that, at the rate you're going, you might well get to a point that something – most likely your liver, but it could be one of all manner of things – goes so wrong that you'll then be in a position in which you really won't be able to drink at all. I'm sure you wouldn't want that, would you? This would be another benefit of cutting down now: it would make it much less likely that you'd ever have to stop completely. I can see you enjoy a drink; I hate to think of you not being able to drink at all.

You're not completely, physically addicted by any means; you don't, I take it, get the shakes if you don't drink. But the danger is that, if you carry on like this, you could well become addicted in that way. Please cut down a bit, so we can stop that happening.

I sent the above words to four GPs I know and braced myself for a tirade of abuse by return of post. There were a couple of severe reprimands issued in decidedly non-medical language, along the lines of, 'take responsibility for your own drinking, you cheeky bastard; how dare you blame us?' Point taken.

Other than that, I was pleasantly surprised; they generally seemed to see what I was getting at, although all of them agreed with some force on one point: they only get about ten minutes with each patient so when exactly are they supposed to get into this stuff? After all, most patients with a drink problem don't come in to talk about their problem with drink, even assuming they recognise they have a problem.

As one of these doctors, a GP in the Cotswolds, put it:

Discussing people's drinking is an opportunistic event – usually not the main reason for the appointment – so it's often easier and quicker to not delve too deeply as most people are either defensive, not interested, or feel you are being judgemental. And frankly, we are so bloody busy, burnt out and overwhelmed that the will to embark upon another issue is pretty low. Also, remember this poor GP of yours has already spent fifteen minutes talking to you and looking at your piles. I expect her motivation is low to then open another can of worms and spend another ten to fifteen minutes talking to you in detail about your drinking while the waiting room backs up.

On the idea of doctors talking about their own drinking to gain the trust of the patient, she had concerns:

I think some people might feel it legitimises their alcohol intake if their doctor reports drinking more than the recommended amount themselves and says they both need to cut down. The patient might just see a green light; it's a fine line.

Another doctor, of Australian heritage, said medics themselves often have a complicated relationship with alcohol:

It means we are not always great at spotting problems in others. Over-50s doctors like me were taught to man up,

*not to bring our problems to work; to do 120 hours a week
without complaining. From medical school onwards, alcohol
was seen as a socially acceptable way of dealing with stress
for doctors. You spend five years at medical school drinking
ten pints, dropping your trousers and pissing in somebody's
flowerbed and then, hey presto, you're a doctor.*

*For GPs, the issue is we have these ludicrous ten-minute
slots to try and sort out incredibly complex problems. As my
trainer used to say, don't go turning over a stone unless you're
prepared to deal with what crawls out underneath. So some
GPs, perhaps deliberately, don't address alcohol, depression,
domestic abuse, homelessness et cetera because they feel
powerless to do much about it in so short a space of time.
And they may also feel a little guilty because of their own
drinking.*

*In the old days you might have a regular GP who you saw
throughout your life, but these days it's very hard to see the
same doctor twice. But there is evidence someone you trust
and respect can make a significant difference by giving you a
firm steer in a single consultation.*

*In terms of your chapter heading, there are thousands
of GPs out there with variable levels of expertise and
engagement when it comes to alcohol. I know GPs who would
be absolutely honest and would say all the things you are
suggesting, and I know others who would deliberately shut
down the consultation.*

*The conversations you wish your doctor had had with you
are all great but, as you know, they may not have made a
difference. What matters is that you're receptive to hearing
them at that particular time and prepared to take some
responsibility yourself. Or, as we say in Australia, sort your
own shit out. It helps if you're surrounded by others going
through the same shit, which is why addiction support groups*

often get better results, but it's often the comment of a doctor that makes you realise you need help.

🍷 🥃 🍺

Funnily enough, I recently came across a great example of this. On a weekend away in a small town somewhere in the home counties, I asked a bloke called Jack, having a smoke outside a pub, if the football was on inside. I was looking for somewhere to watch West Brom in the televised lunchtime match. Jack exclaimed in delight that he, too, was a West Brom fan. My partner rolled her eyes in despair and left us to it.

He was a bit older than me, but younger than he looked. His knowledge of West Brom was not as encyclopaedic as mine, but not far off. He'd been a fan ever since he saw us once on *Match Of The Day* in the seventies. We spent some time reminiscing about happier footballing days before he said, with feeling, 'I'd love to see us play at The Hawthorns one day.' Horrified that this chap had never seen us play at our home ground in half a century supporting us, I promised to take him there.

Our conversation turned to drinking. He told me he wasn't boozing so much anymore after collapsing eighteen months earlier. It turned out that he used to drink enough to make even me wince: six litres of Frosty Jack and a couple of lagers on top of that every day. Frosty Jack, if you're fortunate enough never to have come across it, is a ghastly, super-strong, dirt-cheap cider. I'm not saying it's designed with problem drinkers in mind but, if you were in the business of creating a product for problem drinkers, this is the kind of thing you'd come up with.

'I don't drink it no more,' said Jack.

'How come?'

'Well, when I collapsed, they called an ambulance. When I came round, the ambulance man asked me how much I drank. "No bullshit," he said. "Tell me the truth." So I did, I told him. And he said to me: "If you carry on drinking Frosty Jack, you will die." So I stopped drinking it,' he said with a shrug.

I asked him if anyone else had ever told him he shouldn't drink six litres of Frosty Jack a day. He nodded but said it was something about the way the paramedic put it that made him stop. He still likes a drink, and I very much doubt he's keeping within the safe drinking guidelines, but he's drinking about a third of what he used to. That's no small thing. And all down to a few stern but kind words at the right time from a straight-talking paramedic.

A GP who happens to have been one of the key drinking friends of my teenage years draws a distinction between how drinking and smoking are dealt with:

> I think most GPs have read the evidence on smoking cessation advice. We know that telling someone they should stop because it's bad for you doesn't work. It gets ignored. We know that the best, most successful way, is a package of counselling/support and medication. To my knowledge, this twin approach used for smoking cessation (in reality, often reduction), has never been taught to, or utilised by, GPs in relation to drinking. I've never been taught about how to manage alcohol like this, or ever been aware of any combined counselling and medication support that GPs can provide. I do not know why.

*With smoking, the evidence is that the best type of comment
I can make is to say something like 'cutting down a bit would
be good'. But I have never advised a drinker to reduce a bit. I
realise that I have often looked and seen someone who drinks
a lot and it's never occurred to me they might be addicted
to alcohol (again, ignorance on my part). If they are clearly
drinking too much and putting themselves at risk, then I
generally take a totally different approach and try lines I am
sure you would not like, telling them that it always kills you
somehow – there are many ways but somehow it kills you.*

He, like all the doctors I've spoken to, has been kind enough
to say he'd take on board some of what I'd said. That's less the
case for this GP in Somerset who said:

*Your doctor probably knew that you drank excessively so
didn't need to bring it up at every consultation. My view is
that everyone, particularly those who are intelligent and
educated, have to take personal responsibility for their health
and habit. And until you're ready to do that, nothing any
doctor says would make any difference.*

Harsh, but not entirely unfair.

Vicky and Tim

I came across Vicky Sharpe, a straight-talking South Walian counsellor, via a psychologist friend.

'The bottom line is that alcohol is a legal, reasonably cheap and effective self-medication,' Vicky told me. Her role, as she sees it, is simply to reduce whatever harm alcohol is doing to those she helps. If, in working with them, they agree abstinence is possible, so be it. If moderation, or controlled drinking as she calls it, is the way to go, then that's fine too. Whatever works. Whatever reduces harm.

I've come across all manner of strategies and I'm well beyond judging anyone about anything that works for them. I'm fascinated by the deals drinkers do with themselves. One chap emailed me at work to tell me how he used alcohol as part of an exercise regime. He allowed himself one unit of alcohol for every mile he ran. Bit mad that but, whatever, it works for him.

Someone else I came across weighs himself every morning and if he tops 90 kilos he'll not be drinking until his weight drops below that. There you have it: alcohol as part of both diet and exercise plans.

Vicky is all about whatever works. She put me in touch with someone she'd helped, Tim, a thirty-four-year-old car salesman in Swansea.

I'd been drinking heavily for ten, fifteen years, three or maybe four nights a week. And then it became every night, probably two and a half bottles of wine a night, and I knew I needed to rein it in. I needed something to change, but I knew all along – I'm a realist – that I couldn't stop forever. My brothers all drink; my family all drink; my friends all drink. I just couldn't figure out a way, I couldn't see a possibility of how I was going to get to a stage of never drinking again. Because, either way, it's not going to happen.

You know the only programs out there are like, 'Right, you've got an alcohol problem, so you have to stop completely'. And I just think that isolates a hell of a lot of people because there must be a lot of people out there who would think, 'Well, if I'm going to be told I can never drink again I'm not going to seek help because it's unrealistic'.

Until I met Vicky, I didn't realise there was anyone who would help you without telling you to stop. She said to me, 'Fuck, you're doing 150 units a week'. So we worked out a plan. The idea was to have a period of abstinence and then try to find a routine of drinking, you know, once, maybe twice a week, not spending every single night sitting on the sofa drinking two bottles of wine. So that was the plan we put in place.

We had regular meetings, but it took me a few weeks of talking to her every Tuesday before I started believing I could actually do it.

Vicky, while recognising the importance of three dry months to effect some kind of psychological 'reset', impressed upon Tim that, given his enormous consumption, to stop suddenly might be risky. In cases like his, she'd normally suggest reducing gradually, by around 10 per cent a week. But he insisted that stopping dead – just for a while – was the only way that would work for him. She asked him to monitor any withdrawal symptoms and crack on. He says he wasn't too bad physically, bar 'some sweats and trouble sleeping'. But mentally he had his wobbles.

During that three, four weeks I could quite easily have relapsed at any time, but it was just constantly being able to speak to her that got me through. And then after two months I was thinking I was over half-way there and I could do it.

I didn't have a drink for three months. And now I'm in a position where I'm back to probably two nights a week on Friday, Saturday. So I think that the time not drinking did me a hell of a lot of good, but it's going to be 'til the day I die that I have to keep myself in check. I could slip back into that pattern, yeah, I could. I know I could, so I know I've got to stay on top of it.

I feel great at the moment, and I feel great knowing I can keep it to two days because in my head I'm saying I can't be an alcoholic surely, because I'm able to stick to two days, so that's good. It makes me feel positive.

You could argue, well, would it be better to restrict yourself to three or four days a week and have just a glass or two. But I know that wouldn't work for me. I'll have a bottle and a half on a drinking night now, probably. And that works for me. There's not one universal plan that'll work for everyone. But this works for me. Each to their own.

You may well read Tim's story and despair that he's not got to the bottom of his problem, and it will likely all end in tears. It might, I suppose. But I doubt it. The longer he can sustain this pattern, the greater the chance that the change he's effected will last. I have nothing but admiration for his efforts.

Do I fancy one on a weeknight now? Well, I think I'm over it. My brain does seem to have been reprogrammed. I know the nights I'm going to drink, when I go down and see my brothers or whatever. But if I'm at home, I'm quiet. I do a workout, I'll chill out. And I'm fine with that. I'm absolutely fine with that.

And he's reached a greater understanding of why he drinks in the first place:

It was never a boredom thing, you know. Never was I drinking out of boredom. It's more like whatever I am doing, even just sitting down and watching something, that for some reason I think that if I have a glass of wine, it will be more fun. And it is bollocks. I know it is bollocks because I was watching the US version of The Office. *It's like fucking seven seasons and I can't remember any of it. I drank while I was watching it because I thought it would make it more fun, but it just meant I couldn't remember it. So I now know it's absolute bollocks, this idea that whatever you're doing, whether you're watching a film, whether you're out, whether you're doing this, that or the other, that drinking will make it more fun. You know, you go on holiday and think this is great, but how much better would it be if I was pissed. But it's bollocks.*

Only by stepping back, with Vicky's help, has he found clarity on this. It will help keep him on this path.

I asked Vicky what the secret was in getting through to him, and others like him.

The secret is there is no secret. It's really just about finding the spark in someone and making them believe in themselves.

He wanted to make changes, so we set achievable goals which were flexible. We had an agreed period of abstinence to re-evaluate his relationship with alcohol in general; we worked on some meaningful distractions, and I didn't judge him when he changed his goals. He's pretty typical of his age group. I think a successful intervention looks at the wider picture with a bit of life coaching, a look at his triggers, and some reflection on what alcohol has done and caused in his life. He was very open; I'm really proud of him.

After our chat, Tim tried to sell me a car. I couldn't help him with that, but we did agree to meet up on one of his drinking nights some time and put some wine away together. We'll ask Vicky along too.

My boozing bucket list

Moderation, like all things, needs to be taken in moderation. While I'm very much in favour of us all drinking less, I'm not exclusively about moderation. I still want to go a bit mad every now and then. Here are a few immoderate drinking things I'm still looking forward to doing in my time.

● Every now and then, I still want to go for a quick drink after work, even if I'm finishing at lunchtime. It could be with someone, or some people, I know well, not very well, or not at all. One thing will lead to another and, because (there's no point otherwise) we're having such a brilliant time, the whole escapade will go on far longer than any of us intended. If a marvellous time is had by all then I'm good with this, every now and then.

● Every now and then, should my team win an away game, I still might want to hang around a distant city with a few mates, have several pints and talk about how happy we are and how much we love each other. We may well engage some locals, even fans of the defeated team, in conversation. We'll end up telling them how much we love them too. And how much we all love football. Eventually we'll board a train home, possibly drink a bit more, fall asleep with our mouths open, wake up feeling rubbish but happy, and get ourselves home to bed. I love all this but, as my team don't win away very often, it will only happen every now and then.

● Every now and then, I'll meet up with one or more of my oldest friends, from school or college perhaps. I'm still very close to many of my schoolmates from the day we began our education in January 1972. Ten years or so after the thrilling but bewildering first days of Mrs Timmins' reception class, we were embarking on our drinking careers with just as much excitement and trepidation. Long evenings lay ahead, traipsing around the locale trying to find pubs daft enough to serve underage, bum-fluffed teenagers. I still want to meet up with these now middle-aged gentlemen for long evenings, preferably in one of those same pubs, to drink a lot and discuss what silly buggers we were, and are. Just every now and then.

And there's one other thing I want to do, not every now and then, just the once. I've wanted to do it ever since I was a student in London but somehow never got around to it.

● I'm told by acknowledged experts in the field of excessive drinking that it's actually impossible to do. We'll see. It's called the Circle Line pub crawl. There are thirty-six stations on the London Underground's Circle Line. The idea is to have half a pint of beer at the nearest pub to each of those stations. I make that eighteen pints in total. Apart from the sheer amount of alcohol, it's supposed to be impossible because the need for a wee between stations becomes intolerable. Still, I want to give it a try when I've finished writing this book, with a range of people mentioned herein. Just for the hell of it. It's unnecessary, immature and irresponsible. But, what the heck, such things don't hurt, every now and then.

Forties

As I hit forty, my TV career really took off. The tipping point was presenting *You're Fired*, the companion show to *The Apprentice*. I was also presenting *Match Of The Day 2* as well as *Working Lunch*. The controller of BBC1, Peter Fincham, then had the bright idea of launching a daily magazine show to go out every evening at 7pm on BBC1. We were to pilot this show for three weeks in August 2006 in Birmingham. It was all very stressful, creating a live nationwide television show from scratch to broadcast from a tiny temporary studio located between a Mexican restaurant and a Tesco, next to a canal basin. We came off-air at 7.30, started drinking, and generally carried on long into the night. I'd get up in the morning, run for miles along the canal, work on the show, present it, and go out drinking again. It was like my month in Berlin for the World Cup, except this was Birmingham and there was no international football.

Just like my month in Germany, it was all highly intense and great fun. And the drinking seemed to enhance the whole experience. It's only now that I see fit to ask myself a couple of awkward questions:

1 It was all very well for me to enjoy the benefits of membership of this hard-drinking clique, but what about the colleagues who weren't involved in it? I got to bond and scheme with a good proportion of the production team every night. There were plenty of us – we weren't some elite dining club making all the big decisions – but our group did amount to a clique. So where did that leave the dozens of us who didn't drink at all, for whatever reason, or quite sensibly didn't fancy getting tanked up every night for a month? Sadly, wrongly, they were to some extent out of the loop.

2 How many non-drinkers or light-drinkers ended up having to become heavy drinkers like me for fear of missing out on the professional benefits it doubtless conferred? The answer is, well, I dread to think.

Neither of these questions would have occurred to me at the time, of course. All I was concerned about was making a success of the show, or at least not having it fail spectacularly.

After the first week on-air, nobody seemed quite sure which it was going to be. West Brom had a home game that weekend. As I was walking to the ground, a bloke sitting on a wall with a pint in his hand recognised me and, shaking his head sadly, said, 'Oh Adrian – *The One Show*. Dear oh dear oh dear.' Dispiriting. The audience figures, however, were good enough for this pilot run to be judged a success. *The One Show* was commissioned to run every weeknight, all year round, from July the following year. I left *Working Lunch* after thirteen years to concentrate on this new gig. It worked incredibly well and became a mainstay in the schedule. I also went to cover football's Euros from Vienna and the Olympics in Beijing. At the end of 2008, somebody somewhere worked out that I was the most-watched person on British television that year.

In late 2009 it all started to go a bit sour. It was decreed that the big Friday show every week would be presented by someone else instead of me. I got the hump about this, but the boss stuck to her guns. There wasn't a lot I could do other than suck it up. But then in 2010, ITV came in and offered me a load of money to present their relaunched breakfast show and all their football. Under the circumstances, it wasn't something I could turn down.

I joined them with a huge fanfare from ITV and a big raspberry from the BBC. But *Daybreak*, this new breakfast show, was judged to be a terrible failure with me at the helm and I was soon relieved of my duties on it. My performances presenting football were initially deemed successful. I presented Champions League, International and FA Cup matches. I also covered another Euros, this time in Poland, and World Cups in South Africa and Brazil. But after the latter, in 2014, I was dropped. My twenty-year career in live television was suddenly over.

On top of this heart-stopping, adrenalin-flooding cycle of success, fame and failure, I was also very publicly separating, divorcing and becoming single again.

To describe anything other than a rollercoaster ride as a rollercoaster ride is a cliché. But I use the metaphor to describe my forties because it affords me a very specific image of myself in those years. It looks like this: I'm in one of those jolty rollercoaster videos, my face distorted into various expressions, jumping between fear, joy, trepidation, excitement and other such extremes of emotion. Classically, these videos show a rider clinging onto a big cup of milkshake or coke or something. This they attempt to drink from, even as bits of it fly everywhere. In the video of me I'm holding a pint of Guinness. As I get thrown this way and that on the ride, I'm doing everything in my power to stop the Guinness spilling while trying to take sips of it whenever I can.

This is precisely what my forties felt like.

God, I did some drinking. I presented roughly 600 editions of *The One Show*; I drank after almost every one of those, and to excess after probably 500 of them. There was a green room where we'd linger, often with whichever celebrity we'd had on the show. Having come off-air at 7.30, it wasn't unusual for some of us to still be in there at eleven o'clock. There were also many long evenings in the wine bar next door. And in countless other places all over West London and the West End.

After filming each episode of *You're Fired*, there would be ample to drink in the green room and bar. Later, at ITV, we recorded something called *The Sunday Night Show* every Friday at the same studios, the Riverside in Hammersmith. These recordings would always be followed by plenty to drink in the bar, after which we'd usually go on somewhere else, where we'd remain until far too late.

The punishing hours involved in presenting breakfast television didn't affect my consumption. Getting up at 3.30am and finishing work at 9am was always going to be gruelling, but I assumed I'd be able to get to sleep at lunchtime for a few hours and then carry on with what was left of the day. Sleep proved difficult to come by; the stress of presenting a programme that everybody seemed determined to see fail was probably too much for me. I could barely sleep during the day, or indeed at night. My solution to all this, as with most things, was to drink more – 'to help me sleep,' I told myself. If we went for breakfast after the show, I'd invariably have a couple of Bloody Marys. Caffeine obviously wouldn't aid sleep so, I reasoned, what else was there? A pub across the road from the studios opened early, so a couple of morning pints weren't out of the question either. There were long lunches and evenings out, too.

If I was out in the evening I'd insist on a an early start so I could get to bed at a reasonable hour for my 3.30 alarm call. The problem was that though these evenings started earlier, they generally finished as late as normal. So, sincere as my intentions had been, they only made things worse. I ended up drinking a lot more.

I fully appreciated that I was in the throes of a mid-life crisis, with all the nerve-jangling thrills, spills and bouts of utter despair that entails. I was also single, which didn't help. Clemens Westerhof, a Dutch football coach, despairing of a particularly libidinous group he was in charge of, once said, 'It's not the sex which tires out young players; it's the staying up all night looking for it.' He was bang on there. And while, well into my forties, I could hardly be considered a young player, this definitely applied to me, though without much sex involved; it was more about the drinking. The best thing about being single and on the lookout for someone was that it gave me yet another bloody good excuse to drink.

🍷 🥃 🍺

There was an awful lot of drinking to be done in the business of covering football. I didn't fully realise the extent of it until Roy Keane joined us for the first time to cover a Champions League match in Lisbon. The night before matchday, as usual, we all got together for a meal. Sometimes this would be just a handful of us, but often the entire production team would eat together. If we could find a restaurant big enough, we'd be thirty-strong. On this occasion we were all sitting at one very long table. Roy, I found out, doesn't drink and had a can of coke in front of him. I remember looking up and down the table and seeing he was the only one not drinking alcohol. I noted this for the first time, appreciating that it said something worrying about social norming and our general preoccupation with drink. And then I carried on shovelling it back with my usual dogged enthusiasm.

Before I got relieved of my duties presenting *Daybreak*, these football trips were a blessed escape. We'd fly out to Madrid, Munich, Paris, Milan or wherever the day before. We'd all then meet for lunch or dinner or both, and eat, drink and be merry long into the night. The following day most of us would rise late, maybe have a bit of lunch, and make our way to the stadium to cover the match. After we were done, someone would have arranged somewhere for us to eat, drink and be merry together all over again. We'd make our bleary way back to the UK the following morning.

I suspect the difference between me and my hungover colleagues was that, while most of them would probably ease up on the boozing until their next trip, I'd be out somewhere drinking something with someone or other that very night.

On one of these return flights, a particularly enthusiastic drinker on the team told me how he managed his intake. 'I try to win the week,' he said.

'How do you mean?'

'I try to win the week 4-3; three days drinking and four off it.'

That, I thought, is something I'd not be able to manage.

Even if I'd been unable to drink of an evening because I was working or driving somewhere, I'd usually make strenuous efforts to get to a pub before closing time. In hindsight I find this significant. At the time, it seemed a blameless way of rounding off a long day. Who could question the need for a night cap? And it really wasn't that I was desperately needing a drink on a physical level – I didn't have the shakes or anything remotely like that. It was more like I had an emotional attachment to the idea of it.

Time and again I'd leave Wembley Stadium in a terrible hurry, usually on the back of a taxi bike, desperate to make last orders in my local pub. There I'd glug one or two pints of beer while I chatted to no-one in particular, or just stared into space. I had this compulsion to be there even though it was rarely especially enjoyable. All that rushing just to get a drink that I knew at heart I didn't want, need or enjoy. As an indicator of dependence, it feels as valid as any night on the tiles.

Never once did I consider the monstrous amounts I was drinking and wonder if I was drinking more than was good for me. I never got into trouble, always did a fair bit of exercise and ate well. I don't recall anyone suggesting I might slow down. The closest someone got to that was a television producer and close friend, Paul Connolly. I worked with Paul on *The One Show* and he came with me to *Daybreak* when I left for ITV. We'd regularly have the following conversation when I turned up at the office before 5am.

'Big night last night?' he'd ask.

'Nah, non-drinking night,' I'd reply.

'How much did you drink then?'

'Two pints of Guinness and half a bottle of wine.'

'OK, got it. Proper non-drinking night.'

The point being, of course, that there was never such a thing as a genuine non-drinking night, as defined as a night without, you know, any drinking at all. Two pints of beer and half a bottle of wine was the closest I came to zero so, as Paul spotted, it had become my zero.

After I got the boot from ITV, not much changed on the drinking front. In terms of my rollercoaster video, it would show the rollercoaster crashing to a halt. I'd then be seen getting up and walking away, supping what was left in my glass, on my way to buy another pint.

Forties drinks scorecard

● CONSUMPTION

I can't see how, on average, I was drinking any less than **100 units a week**. Over the course of my fifth decade as a whole, this was in total roughly the equivalent of 520 bottles of wine, more than 24,000 pints of Guinness, or 50,000 shots. Horrifying.

● BORING BITS

Another restaurant in another European city with some really interesting people. One night blurs into the next but I can't say it was ever boring. The craic wasn't always of Champions League standard, but it was rarely far off. Back home, the stress of working on what was perceived as a failing show was awful. Day after day I'd drink a couple of pints just to calm the anxiety a bit. At that point I'd feel OK; the medicine seemed to work. When I went beyond those two pints, which I did most nights, the anxiety would fade into boredom. I was bored with the same feeling of chronic fatigue, worsened by alcohol, night after night in some bar or restaurant or club, having eaten and drunk more than I wanted, needed, or enjoyed. I'd stand around unsteadily, wondering how I was going to pull out of whatever conversation I was in and get myself into bed and then up again a few hours later to go and do it all over again.

● PROPORTION OF DRINKS WANTED/NEEDED/ENJOYED

60 per cent.

I was no longer able to distinguish between these three things. When the craic was good, I wanted and enjoyed every drink. When I was losing my mind with stress, I didn't enjoy anything. At those times I didn't have a clue what I wanted or needed in life, apart from a drink that is, which was something I told myself I always wanted or needed or enjoyed, no matter what.

There would be times when I was so depressed I could barely put one foot in front of the other. Sitting at home staring at a wall was unbearable. I'd walk across the little park next to my place to the shops. I'd move very slowly. Everything felt like it was in slow motion; every blink of my eye and each breath I took. Only two things alleviated these feelings, and then only temporarily. One was a run, the other was a drink. Then, one Sunday morning, the running stopped working. I ran as fast as I could around Gunnersbury Park and felt no better at the end than I had at the start.

A drink or two, however, never stopped working. And it was only, literally, a drink or two that I needed. I suppose I was blessed that that was all it took. It rarely killed the misery completely, which often came back worse or less bad the following morning; but it was enough to afford me some relief, to reset, and then try again.

I know now, as I knew then, that this was an unsatisfactory state of affairs, but there you go. At least I knew when to stop on these occasions; I rarely cracked on and had, by a heavy drinker's standard, an absolute skinful. Perhaps if a skinful was what it took to get the relief I needed, it would have been a skinful I'd drink. In which case I'd have been in grave trouble. I might be just lucky that I didn't need that much; I didn't need to achieve a state of oblivion. Or perhaps from somewhere I had the awareness that to have drunk to oblivion at these times would have risked truly catastrophic outcomes. I know not where this level of self-control came from, but I thank God for it.

A pint under a hawthorn tree

During the COVID-19 lockdown, the power of social norming was there for us all to see. If we got the feeling everyone was respecting the lockdown rules, we'd be more inclined to observe them ourselves. Conversely, if we sensed they were being flouted by lots of people, we'd be more inclined to get out there and do likewise.

It's the same with drinking. Because we're encouraged to believe that everybody drinks too much, just like us, we're more inclined to do the same. A reminder: most drinkers do drink 14 units or less a week.

None of which changed the fact that one sunny locked-down day I couldn't stop thinking about a pint. Earlier that day I'd driven past a pub near me out of which I saw two blokes wheeling a mobile beer-tap thing. I logged this information. I'd not had a pint of draught beer in nearly two months. Sitting at my desk trying to write a book about drinking less, I'd been quite unable to concentrate; all I could think of was the possibility of a draught beer. Every time I closed my eyes, all I could see was condensation forming on pipes.

I arranged to meet a friend for a walk. Accidentally on purpose, I had us wander in the direction of the pub. I found the experience so profoundly enjoyable that I immediately wrote it down, like a diary entry.

'Where are we going?' he asks.

'Oh, erm, I think they're selling draught beer outside the Duchess,' I say.

And, as if by magic, suddenly we are there.

There is Peroni and there is Guinness. I get us a Guinness each and, abiding by the pourer's instructions not to linger, we repair to a nearby park. We sit at each end of a rickety bench beneath a hawthorn tree, and carefully remove the lids from our plastic pint glasses. With slow reverence we take our sips. We sit quietly chatting for half an hour or so and give thanks for this simple pleasure.

And then we make our respective ways home.

That pint was a beautiful thing. It's drinks like that one – and it was just the one – that I cherish. I always want to be able to access this simple joy. This is why I'm trying to drink less, so I don't mess myself up and make a pint with a mate under a hawthorn tree a thing of the past.

What I learned from Lee Mack (or, 'It could all be a giant con')

Lee Mack is a brilliant comedian of my acquaintance, and someone with strong views on alcohol. His parents were publicans; both died in their fifties as a result of their alcohol intake. His brother also had serious alcohol issues. Lee decided to cut down on his drinking a lot, but then decided to stop altogether because he was persuaded that the whole thing was, essentially, a con.

Though my family history is not as extreme, Lee and I grew up with, and into, similar drinking patterns.

I was classed as a 'normal' drinker, I suppose. But, you know, what is normal? In my 30s I would open a bottle of wine with dinner and finish it in front of the telly. So I'd have a bottle of wine. That would be fairly normal in today's society from what I see around me. You know, I'm not doing that every night but it's also fair to say that some nights I was opening that second bottle. You know what I mean.

Yes, I know what he means. I also knew what he meant when he said:

> *You know that feeling of sitting down with a pint of lager after a long day? You sit outside the pub in the sunshine at six o'clock; you take that first mouthful of beer and you go, 'Aaaah'. You know that instant feeling. It feels great.*

Yes, all deliciously familiar. But then came the bit I hadn't thought of:

> *The thing is, it's medically proven that alcohol doesn't instantly get in your bloodstream. It takes 10 minutes, according to the Institute for Alcohol Abuse. So that instant feeling of relaxation cannot be the alcohol, because it's not in your bloodstream. Something else is going on.*

Yes, it must be. I wondered why it was that I felt just as good after my first sip, even if it was from a can of alcohol-free beer I got out of the fridge, rather than Guinness. So what is going on?

I went straight to the top for an answer to this, from his eminence David Nutt, professor of neuropsychopharmacology and author of a brilliant book, *Drink? The New Science of Alcohol and Your Health*.

The prof told me that alcohol does indeed take between ten and twenty minutes to get into the brain, so to that extent Lee's theory holds true. But then he added this caveat: 'Over time people learn to associate the brain effects with the state. So that the taste of alcohol – which is usually aversive to start with –

becomes more and more liked, as it gets associated with the later predicted positive effects of alcohol.'

So, in a nutshell, David's view is that we have a substance which we, at first, generally don't like the taste of. Then, once we've experienced positive mental effects from the alcohol, we acquire a taste for it. And eventually, in anticipation of these nice feelings, the very taste of alcohol can trick us into thinking we're already feeling its pleasurable effects.

Which means there *is* a bit of a con going on here somewhere. It's Lee's view that alcohol confuses us about what it is that is making us feel good.

Let's say it's the first time you've sat down after a long day. You've got a nice cold drink and you're not working anymore. You're already in a better mood than you were at work, but because you've got the booze in, you immediately think, Oh I'm feeling good because of the booze.

So the booze gets the credit. Alcohol, take a bow.

Likewise, you've been at a party and you go, 'I had a great time last night; I was pissed, had a great time'. So you immediately assume you had a great time because you were pissed, as opposed to you had a great time with your mates having a laugh but you just happened to be drinking at the same time. It feels that way because you often associate drinking with the enjoyable thing you're also doing at the time. In the same way, if every time you took a sip of lager I whacked you on the head with a hammer, you'd associate the taste of lager with pain and stress. It's the association with what you're doing. I just came to think it was all a con.

I can't quite dismiss all the positive effects of alcohol as a complete con. But Lee's right, if only in that it depends on what you believe: if you believe, as I always have, that alcohol is your key to the door of joy then that will become your truth; if you believe, like Lee, that it's all a con, then you'll soon see straight through it.

For my part, I think the truth, boringly, is somewhere between the two. But ever since I spoke to Lee I've leaned more to his way of thinking than my own.

As well as being annoyed at what he sees as the con of it all, Lee despairs at the extent to which the 'blame' for drinking issues is laid at the door of the individual rather than the industry which devotes itself to selling us the stuff.

In your documentary I noticed that you were always saying, 'Am I drinking too much?' or 'Am I a normal drinker? And if I'm not, what is it about me that makes me drink like this?' All this 'What is it about me?' is what the industry has made us all believe.

If a man knocked on your door and started selling your kid heroin and your kid got addicted, you'd want to strangle the bloke selling the heroin. You wouldn't go, 'What is it about my son that's made him addicted to this stuff?' You wouldn't be asking that question. I always wonder why it is with alcohol that we let the suppliers get away without taking more of the blame.

I've wondered as much myself, on more than one occasion. There's another area Lee and I generally agree on. When we talk about the notion of 'alcoholism' as a 'disease' all the nodding in agreement makes our necks hurt.

I just don't buy the idea of alcoholism as a disease even though I suppose I should think that way because my parents died of it. I should want to believe that. The problem with saying that I don't believe the disease theory is that people then automatically assume that you believe in the opposite theory – essentially that we all only have ourselves to blame. But I don't believe that either.

What I believe in is a third option, which is simply that it's a highly addictive drug. You ask anyone why they drink and they will tell you all sorts: they like the taste, it's relaxing, it's a laugh, it makes them more socially confident etc., etc. But the answer that is probably the most true is one that is hardly ever given – that they're addicted to it. Of course they are, it's highly addictive. And if you take it, you are going to get addicted to it to different degrees. And how addicted you get is not in your control.

Now that's the bit where I tend to disagree with Lee; I wouldn't be writing this book if I didn't. I agree that we're all addicted to a degree, but I believe you can, in most cases, if you choose to, have some control over the extent of your addiction, if only by being aware of the challenge and appreciating that the more you drink, the more addicted you're likely to become. And the opposite applies too: drink less and you'll probably become less dependent.

That said, Lee definitely has a point when he says that:

Some people need a pint, and that's enough. Some people need three or four pints to satisfy their addiction to this addictive drug. Some people need ten. Some people need it from the minute they wake up to the minute they go to bed. And that's the bit that's not in your control. Yet people say, Well, if it's not a disease, why do some people have their lives ruined by it, and some don't?

But if you saw three people stuck in quicksand, one up to his neck, one to his waist and one to his ankles, you wouldn't start asking why it was that one of them was almost buried and the others less so. You'd just say get out of the fucking quicksand; it's the quicksand that's the danger, not the people. The bottom line is that the quicksand, like alcohol, is the problem.

I just don't agree with the word alcoholic; the problem is, if you have the word alcoholic, who's going to go and get help if the only way of dealing with it is to admit you are one; that you have a disease you're going to have the rest of your life and you're different to most other members of society who are 'non-alcoholics'? Who's going to put their hands up and say, yes that's me?

Why does it have to be binary? If you smoke five a day, you're addicted to cigarettes to the extent of five a day; if you smoke ten, you're addicted to the extent you need to smoke ten. There's no set number of cigarettes it takes for you to be smoking for someone to decide your smoking is now out of control and say, from now on we'll call you a smokerholic.

There's not a point where you change the word to something else. The only drug we do that for is booze. If you take heroin, you're a heroin addict, or you're not. Anyone who takes heroin at all regularly would be regarded by society as an addict, but never as a heroinoholic. Anybody who smokes fairly regularly would be called an addict; anyone who does any drugs, even if it's in control, would be called to some degree an addict. But with the booze, because everyone does it – including the police, doctors and judges – they have this word alcoholic to use, so they can say, I'm not that person.

He's right: 'I'm not that person', is an expression of what psychologists call 'othering'. This 'I'm-not-as-bad-as-that-person' mantra of self-justification is rife in all kinds of situations. In driving, tax avoidance, fidelity, criminality, you name it; we can always point to someone worse than us. But with drinking it is right at the heart of the problem, aided and abetted by this idea of 'alcoholism' as a 'disease' that you either have or you don't.

This idea of this thing called alcoholism as an illness has obviously come from a good place, and I have total empathy with that; the aim of taking the blame away from the individual, the drinker. But, ironically, in doing so it kind of puts all the emphasis on that individual rather than the pushers – the alcohol industry. Can you imagine how we'd all feel if a smoker got lung cancer and the cigarette companies said, 'It's not our fault; that person must have sensitive lungs'?

Having lost his parents to alcohol, seen his brother suffer too, and quietly drunk to excess himself before changing that, Lee's earned the right to have a view, and it's one I find compelling, even if it means that in drinking less rather than nothing I'm still falling for the con.

I completely understand why people get addicted to booze, because I was addicted to it; not to the point where my life was going wrong, but I was addicted to it. I now realise it's a con. And it doesn't do the things you think it's doing.

For me, logic dictates that if you can allow yourself to be conned by the first drink of the evening making you feel great, then you can also be conned about the latter part of the night when the alcohol HAS kicked in. You could be dancing, chatting, laughing and so on and assume it's because of the booze. But I don't think it is.

🍷 🥃 🥛

As with just about every subject on earth, there are academic research papers available on this. I came across one by four Hungarian academics entitled 'Alcohol and Placebo: The Role of Expectations and Social Influence', published in the *International Journal of Mental Health and Addiction*. As with most academic papers, it is written in a language which non-academics, like me, struggle with. It's written in English, but lots of it might as well have been in Hungarian for all I understood.

But here's what I could glean: they gave 136 people rum and cokes to drink. Some of these were made with real rum, some with a non-alcoholic alternative. It was established in a separate experiment that the two drinks were indistinguishable in taste. The participants then drank these rum and cokes, real or fake, in a variety of situations. Some drank alone, others in groups. Some were told which of the two they were drinking; others weren't. And some were misinformed: they were told they were drinking alcohol when they weren't, and vice versa.

This is some of what the researchers believe they established:

> *It seems that it is enough for people to believe they have consumed alcohol to feel inebriated. The aim of the study was also to clarify the role of group conditions in the placebo effect. Comparing the results of the individual and group settings, regardless of the alcohol content of the consumed cocktail, a social atmosphere intensified the effects of alcohol consumption.*

In other words, if you believe there is alcohol in your drink then you'll most likely feel the effect of it whether there was alcohol in it or not. And this is particularly the case if you're drinking in a social situation rather than alone.

To summarise, the effect of alcohol can only be partly explained by ethanol [alcohol], as several other factors – mainly social processes, suggestions and expectations – play an important role in how individuals become inebriated.

So, more evidence for Lee that there's a bit of a con going on here somewhere.

Eighty-odd years before these four Hungarians – Bodnar, Nagy, Cziboly and Bardos – were reaching these conclusions, not so far away in Yugoslavia, Rebecca West was writing her mighty doorstep of a travelogue, *Black Lamb and Grey Falcon*. Listening to Lee Mack talking, and reading about this research in Hungary, a line in West's book came to mind. Miraculously, leafing through the 1,150 pages of my copy, I found it.

West, ruminating on the nature of Turkish people, makes all sorts of lazy generalisations. On Muslims' eschewal of alcohol, she says the following:

The reward for total abstinence from alcohol seems, illogically enough, to be the capacity for becoming intoxicated without it.

While I flinch at the unmistakeable sound of an Islamo-phobic dog whistle there, she inadvertently gets at something important. Those of us who speak of the societal benefits of alcohol, such as its value as a social lubricant and so on, need to address a couple of awkward questions: are we really saying that people in alcohol-free societies don't socially cohere as well as we do (if we do)? And do they not experience love, joy, laughter and all the good things every bit as keenly as we do? In fact, is alcohol – or any other chemical – actually necessary in order to feel something like intoxication?

Probably not, would be Lee Mack's view I'm sure, because alcohol is a con. The more I think about it, the more I think he may be right.

∇ ∇ ∇

Interestingly, it wasn't complete abstinence that led Lee to his conclusions; it was his early attempts at moderation.

When I first thought about cutting down or stopping boozing, I made a deal with myself that I would start every night with two drinks that were ice cold and no-alcohol, usually zero-alcohol lager. And after them I could have whatever alcoholic drinks I liked, and with no limit. I found that by the time I'd finished those first two drinks I was just not as interested in booze as I was at the start of the evening. Why would I be when, without it, I was still relaxed, refreshed and having a laugh? Also, two pints of any liquid is enough; it's only the addictive element that makes you want more.

If there is one single tip to take away from this book, it is this one. It's worked so well for me that I've given it a name – the *Lee Mack Rule of Two*. The expression is *To Do a Mack*. I hope that one day the words, 'Oh, an alcohol-free please – I'm Doing a Mack', will be commonly heard in pubs across the country.

Something
Roy Keane said

Roy Keane once said something to me about drinking that really hit home. If someone else had said it, there wouldn't have been the same impact, somehow. I suppose it's the difference between being tackled by Roy Keane and being tackled by anyone else who's ever played the game.

If you're not into football, all you need to know about Roy is that he's one of the greatest players ever. He coupled huge talent with insane levels of drive and determination. On the pitch and off, he's always been a captivating, not to say occasionally terrifying, presence.

By the time I got to know him, working together covering football, he'd not touched alcohol in more than ten years. This didn't seem to affect his social life; he was always great company when we were away on our travels around Europe. Our colleague Tony Pastor and I did an awful lot of drinking as the three of us wandered around Barcelona, Warsaw, Munich or wherever. We had some great days, at least Tony and I did. I'm assuming Roy did too. Well, put it like this: he never told us he didn't and he's not one to keep such thoughts to himself.

I'd popped in to see him for a cup of tea at his place in Altrincham. It was during Lent, so I wasn't drinking. (I'm noticing, by the way, just how many of my insights into my own drinking came at times when I wasn't drinking.) Roy and I got on to the subject, and he, as I remember it, said something like this:

> *The problem is there's always a reason to drink. If you've had a good day, you want a drink. Or a bad day. Or even just a boring day. A wedding's a good reason to drink and, even more so, funerals. If you've won a match, or lost a match, or had a row with someone or are getting on well with someone. If you're going out, or staying in. Or whatever. There's always a reason to drink.* *

I wouldn't argue with Roy on that. Then again, I'm loath to argue with Roy about anything. But no need here anyway, because he's 100 per cent right.

---

* I thought I'd better run this chapter past Roy before I sent it to the publisher. He came back with something interesting, a correction actually. He pointed out that he never said these things were a 'reason' to drink. He said they were an 'excuse' to drink. Again, he's bang on: yes, these things are an excuse, not a reason to drink. And it's doubtless significant that he used one word, but I remembered another. So, to be clear, what the great Roy Keane said is that 'the problem is there's always an excuse to drink'. How true, how painfully true.

Her name is Marisa and she is a moderator

Marisa is a freelance journalist in her thirties. I came across her through the psychologist who helped her to moderate her drinking, Shahroo Izadi. Marisa rarely drank a massive amount in one go, but she drank so regularly that she came to feel it was getting out of hand.

I was working for a start-up, and it was completely full on. I was drinking a lot, and often. I was never drinking at an hour I felt uncomfortable with, but I realised that drinking had kind of become the solution to everything. So, if I had a bad day, I was going to the pub; if I had a good day, I was going to the pub; if I had a day off, I was going to go to the pub. In the end I saw that whenever I wasn't actually working, I was always drinking.

It had become that it felt like alcohol was almost essential for survival, and to reward myself with, and to kind of medicate myself with. At that time, every day it seemed to be providing everything for me. There were times when I got really drunk, and there was all that chaos and calamity that comes with drinking too much. That was pretty common; one night I got all my belongings nicked. But in general, the problem was the frequency with which I was drinking.

Essential. She says drinking felt essential to her in every way. I've been there. Essential. The more I hear anyone use that word in relation to the role of drinking in their life, the more I think it's a strong indicator of trouble.

Maybe it is the key question that should appear on all those questionnaires about your relationship with alcohol: do you consider the taking of alcohol to be a) unimportant, b) important or c) essential to your enjoyment of life. If you're answering c), then I think we need to talk.

It is one thing to enjoy drinking, or to feel it enhances your enjoyment of life. That's fine. If you think to some extent it helps you get through life, that's sub-optimal but, in my view, just about OK. However, if you feel it is nothing less than essential – as I did for an awfully long time – then I think alcohol has taken control of you and you need to turn it round, and show alcohol that you're the one in charge.

That's certainly what Marisa felt she had to do, which was never going to be a walk in the park given how central drinking had become in her life.

I could leave my office and be in the pub within about ten minutes, and that first drink would make me feel different. And I couldn't stop chasing that feeling. I remember thinking, how can I not be in the pub? How can I not have a drink? I remember it being such an impossibility in my head. But it is do-able.

Interestingly, Marisa never counted how many units she was, or is, drinking. This rather flies in the face of my contention that doing so is essential to the whole endeavour of trying to drink less, but I'll let her off.

I'd have to think and kind of work it out for you, but I've always stayed well clear of even trying to kind of understand that stuff. When you're like I was, you stay away from any of the actual realities of the harm it's causing you.

What she managed to do, without the unit number-crunching I put myself through, or anything like John Robins' calendar-marking, was to work on changing her way of thinking.

I didn't believe I needed to stop; I just needed to have a different relationship with wine and what it meant in my life. Basically, I needed to work out why I drank and when; it kind of became about ring-fencing the times when I enjoy drinking. I realised that being in a pub at last orders on a Monday evening is a miserable place to be. Whereas Friday night with my mates in the pub was a place I really wanted to be.

Ring-fencing; nicely put. It's another way of expressing what I'm always banging on about: working out which drinks you actually want and enjoy and sticking to them. But identifying these important wheres, whens and whats is only half the battle; to get there, a lot of hard-wired habits have to change.

I had to stop getting to like six o'clock and emailing a few friends who I always knew would want to drink with me. I realised I'd have to curtail the sending of that email saying, 'Fancy a quick drink?' because it would never be a quick drink.

Marisa credits much of her success in changing her ways to Shahroo Izadi, a psychologist who helped her learn to treat herself with the same kindness she might afford a close friend. So, for example, if my dearest friend was drinking at the level I was drinking at, I'd probably suggest it would be a good idea for them to cut down a bit. I wish it hadn't take so long to give myself this advice.

It's the kind of wise counsel Marisa started giving – and taking – herself.

> *Instead of the pub, I'd go home and have a bath and do all these other relaxing things. I suddenly felt fantastic. Oh my God, I'd wake up completely clear-headed and think, 'God, the things I could do'. I look back at those days and I just remember the hangovers and the existential crises that came with the hangovers. And the time I wasted and the money I wasted, and I just don't want to go back to those days.*

> *I still very much enjoy a drink and I very much enjoy being in a pub and still look at alcohol as some kind of remedy, but I just try to think a bit more long-term. So instead of just being like, bang, this will fix me now, I just trained myself to think a bit, actually. Like if I do this tonight, how will I feel tomorrow and then how will I feel tomorrow night? So, often I now have three or four nights without a drink.*

Not that there aren't challenges. These she deals with by identifying them, trying to deal with them and, crucially, if she slips up, forgiving herself.

> *Being at a friend's house is always kind of a dodgy place for a moderate drinker. People think they're being polite when they top your glass up the minute it's empty. And you feel you're*

being impolite if you don't drink it. Those social pressures on drinking are very real still, and that's always a tricky space for me because you can get to somebody's house at lunchtime and you're there till ten o'clock and it's all been just booze.

This is where Marisa has to put Shahroo Izadi's ideas, about being as kind to herself as she would be to a friend, into action.

The days I tend to drink more, I think I kind of give myself a free pass on those a bit because they're only occasional. And I know, yes, I'm probably over my limit of units or whatever, but it's not like I'm still in the pub every night of the week. If I was, I'd be worried. But now I'm not, so it's fine.

In other words, be kind to yourself by forgiving yourself. Just because you've gone a bit mad one night, there's no need for drama. Don't beat yourself up. It's happened before, it'll happen again, but mostly you're doing OK. That'll do.

Marisa also points out it helps to have a partner who doesn't drink much.

My boyfriend doesn't drink loads, and I have wondered what I would be like if I met a really heavy drinker. He's helped me. The reality is I'm not gonna open a bottle of wine for one glass if he doesn't want any. And he'll always know when he's had enough. I guess it takes away that normalisation of just a bottle of wine always being in the fridge, always on hand.

Neither finding a nice boyfriend nor a way of being kinder to yourself is necessarily straightforward of course. Marisa also stresses the psychological spadework you need to put in.

I think you've got to understand why you're drinking too much. You know, there's a reason. And if you can understand that reason, you can start to unlock some of your own behaviours; you can start to understand when and why you're going for it with drinking. If you can work that out, it's all more likely to work in the long term.

It's worked for her; she's nearer where she wants to be but still confesses to having her needs.

I rarely want to go into a pub and have one drink; I always like two. Once you've had that first one, that longing for the second is still there. But now I know that two is enough. And then I'm on my way.

To which I say, good work, Marisa. But she finishes by making a point that pulls me up short; something that I must admit I'd never thought of. She says that drinking moderately – part of which involves considering the consequences of drinking too much – in a sense runs counter to the advice that we're always getting these days about the importance of living in the moment.

I must admit I miss the feeling of kind of complete freedom in life. I know in most ways drinking is pointless, but it can give you that feeling of being completely in the moment; that true – or maybe false – feeling of being carefree. And I always felt like anything could happen in those moments; I could meet anyone to go anywhere and there was all this excitement. And it was also about being present, and I missed that.

I missed that because I think drinking moderately is about not being in the present, because you're having to recognise how you're going to feel in the future.

When I write about drinking, I talk about how I had this slightly ridiculous alter ego called Shelby who would come out when I was drunk. She was the version of me who was confident enough to say all the things I'm not confident enough to say when I haven't had a bottle of wine. And I miss that feeling of being alive, of feeling anything could happen tonight.

Yes, yes, yes. We both enthusiastically agree with each other in recognition of that feeling, before catching ourselves – and reminding ourselves that the feeling itself is just a fallacy. I say, very much as if I'm trying to convince myself, that there's got to be a way of feeling that alive without actually drinking.

Yes, exactly. And I think that's a really good point, isn't it? What are you really missing anyway? If I'm being how I really want to be when I'm drunk, then at least I know how I want to be. And that's why it's important to work out what you use booze for, and then you can find a better way of getting there without it.

Shahroo and kindness

Shahroo Izadi, the psychologist who helped Marisa get a grip on her drinking, is the author of a book called *The Kindness Method*. Its inspiration was her experience of food addiction and yo-yo dieting. But its message – life is stressful, be kind to yourself and then learn how to strengthen your willpower so that you can sustain motivation for the long haul – applies to all kinds of addictions. As a specialist in behavioural change, Shahroo has helped drinkers of all kinds.

She starts by working out how much they drink, as well as how, when and why they do it. Her trick for getting honest answers to these questions is to try to take the shame out of it.

Invariably, they feel judged. So I think taking the judgement away from their alcohol consumption is vital. Otherwise once they come to see quite how much they are drinking they might start beating themselves up about it. If you're not careful you can increase their negative vision of themselves before you can do anything about it. So when I'm talking about the number of drinks they're having, or even the number of drinks they want to cut out, I try to take the judgement out; I get them to imagine we're talking about squash.

She's so right. When anyone asks you about your drinking you feel like you're in the dock. And since no-one's asked you to swear on a bible to tell the truth, and you may be quietly ashamed of the truth, why would some dishonesty not creep in?

I advance to Shahroo my lovingly developed theory that the trick of moderation is first to identify the drinks you really enjoy; the ones which make all the difference to you. All you then need to do is carry on enjoying them and cut the rest out. Simple, really. She makes assenting noises but then says something which pulls me up short:

But what about if you're just drinking for oblivion?'

That's an excellent question and, absurdly, not one I'd really considered. Because, whatever I drink for, it's not oblivion. Don't get me wrong, I've achieved oblivion in my time but very rarely since I was a teenager. I grew out of this need to get absolutely smashed. If you do feel this need, then I suppose moderation is going to be trickier for you. Perhaps I've been able to moderate successfully because I've managed to get what I want out of alcohol before reaching oblivion. If it's oblivion you're after, you're plainly going to struggle to find it if you're drinking less.

Either way, Shahroo says the key is to get drinkers to project themselves further forward than the moment when they're shouting up the next drink.

The problem is that so many people drink not to care. And alcohol as a drug is very good at that; it's very efficient at making you stop caring. It puts drinkers in the moment when they want nothing more than to meet their short-term needs.

In other words, the one thing you need them to do – to consider some consequences – is exactly what alcohol tends to stop you doing.

So, I try to identify why they're drinking, because diminishing returns are a real thing. When I ask people when it was during the evening they really enjoyed the alcohol and it was really doing something for them, they invariably say it's the second drink, not the seventh.

For me, it's the first drink, but never mind. To make her point she's devised a clever exercise.

I did a chart for a client recently with three columns on it. In the first column there was one glass of wine. In the next column there was space to write the positives of having that glass of wine. Then in the third column you could write the negatives. Against the one glass of wine there was plenty in the pros column and nothing in the cons. And the same for glass number two. But with each additional glass the pros column got emptier as the cons column filled up. At the bottom, when we'd finished with the wine, I put 'following day'. Next to it the pros column was empty.

In the spirit of this, I made a chart for a typical night, back in the day, meeting a friend in our local at 6pm on, say, a Tuesday. It was a bit of a shock, seeing it set out on paper.

1. Guinness	Pros: Pure pleasure; looking forward to another.	Cons: None.
2. Guinness	Pros: Bit less pleasure but still nice.	Cons: Starting to feel peckish so trough some crisps.
3. Guinness	Pros: The black stuff is still slipping down.	Cons: Feeling a bit woozy.
Switch to 4. Red wine	Pros: It's OK. Change is as good as a rest.	Cons: Starting to struggle to get to the bottom of the glass.
5. Red wine (2nd glass from bottle)	Pros: None really; though it keeps me in the pub, which is possibly good.	Cons: Really don't like the taste; conversation waning. Also, I've eaten so many crisps, nuts and whatnot that my hands and lips are as greasy as the rim of my glass and I can feel my heartburn revving up.

6. More red wine, another bottle having been ordered.

Pros: None, other than a feeling of school-night mischief, which is nice.

Cons: Lots. Now feeling really full, bored and thinking about what a vast amount of something I'll shortly be eating in front of the TV at home.

7. Guinness – my mate ordered one on the way back from the toilet.

Pros: refreshing, I suppose, after all that wine, but otherwise no positives at all.

Cons: feeling full to the brim, groggy and wishing I'd left after the second pint at the latest.

I go home, eat vast doorstep sandwiches and crisps in front of the TV, and eventually blubber my way to bed.

In the morning, looking back.

Pros: just as in Shahroo's client's case, there aren't any.

Cons: Plenty. I'd feel a bit plain and generally quite overwhelmed by the physical and financial cost of it all, and the general pointlessness. Usually.

But, but, but, that 'usually' is key here. I totally get Shahroo's purpose in setting this exercise, and it's a really useful thing to do. But my problem is, or was, this: in truth, there were the odd evenings when the craic was suddenly very good and a fabulous night out unfolded. Someone interesting and funny might turn up out of the blue and, all of a sudden it would be closing time on a weeknight and we'd had an unexpectedly marvellous time.

If that was the case, in the morning my assessment might have looked like this:

- Pros: had a cracking night; it was like the old days; felt young again; forged new friendships and renewed old ones. Everyone involved lovingly filed away the shared memory of a great evening, to be fondly recalled for days, weeks, months and even years.

- Cons: well, none really. Slight hangover perhaps.

If you drink most nights, and most of those nights turn out this good, then I feel more pity for you than envy. If it's always so brilliant, and if you're convinced that copious alcohol is key to it, you're going to have a hell of a job cutting down. But I just can't believe drinking can be that good that often. It certainly wasn't for me. The trouble is that when they do happen, those great nights are *really* great and that, pardon the pun, is what's so intoxicating about them. This leads to a couple of bits of stinking thinking, which I've certainly been guilty of.

Firstly, I told myself it was the alcohol which made it all possible. I was convinced that if I hadn't had that skinful the craic wouldn't have been anything like as good. If I hadn't been drinking at all, by my logic, I wouldn't have been there in the first place. And if I'd stuck at a drink or two then it wouldn't have been half as good.

Secondly – and this is the real killer – I've come to understand that I was only there in the first place for fear of missing out on one of those rare cracking nights. They did happen, for sure, but they certainly weren't the norm. But so precious were they that, instead of bailing out early, I'd often keep drinking on the majority of evenings – the boring, pointless ones – in the (usually vain) hope that one of those great nights would materialise.

This kind of 'alcoholic FOMO' led me into pouring an enormous amount of unwanted, unenjoyed and unneeded booze into my system.

Bearing all this in mind, here is my chart for the odd week-night out these days:

1. Guinness (pint)	Pros: absolutely love it.	Cons: none, apart from the two units I'm 'spending' of my weekly limit.
2. Guinness (pint)	Pros: love it almost as much.	Cons: getting a bit fuzzy towards the bottom of this one. Half a pint would have been enough, actually.

And then I go home; that'll do me.

| **The following morning:** | Pros: Really enjoyed it at the end of a long day. It was good to catch up with whoever, or sit on my own and read, or just stare into space. And feel in control. | Cons: none. Another reminder, should I have needed it, that I always want to be able to do this. |

There's another one of Shahroo's techniques I really like. She encourages her clients to write a list of all the reasons they might regret drinking so much.

All the reasons they don't want to be drinking; all the reasons they came to see me; all the ways they know they are going to feel tomorrow. And all the things they might regret about what they say or how they behave; how sick they might feel and how they might remedy that state with probably quite unhealthy food. And that's going to have a knock-on effect on their mental health and whether they go to the gym and all these things. I tell them to write these things down, keep them on their phone, and put an alert on to have a look at that list when they go to the loo at the party. Because they will not be remembering that stuff at that moment, partly because of the mind-altering effect of alcohol, but also because they want to forget.

Here's my list, which I may or may not have the presence of mind to squint at, myopically, on my phone as I stand at a urinal, swaying slightly, too many drinks into a night out:

- Are you really enjoying yourself?

- Did you enjoy that last drink?

- Are you looking forward to your next drink?

- If there was a button to get yourself zapped home in a trice right now, would you press it?

I think that on at least half of the nights out in my life my answers to the above questions would have been as follows: suppose so, not really, no, yes. What a waste.

At the races

One day, towards the end of the last century, I was at Newbury Races making a radio documentary about gambling. I was there with a successful professional gambler, not a species I'd come across before. He dressed and talked like an accountant, perhaps a partner in a trendy, up-and-coming provincial practice. I liked him.

These were the days when, in theory, the only way to place a tax-free bet was to go to a race meeting and use an on-course bookmaker. Accordingly, this chap, having assiduously studied the form and identified his winners, would travel to racecourses to make sizeable bets. He didn't make many bets, so the ones he did place had to be worthwhile. Not being born yesterday, I put my relatively paltry twenty quid on the same horse as him and it duly won. After we'd collected our winnings he said, 'Let me tell you something: you'll always remember the name of that horse, and the odds too, probably. You never forget the winners.'

Getting on for a quarter of a century later I can tell you that he was right. The horse was called Kato and he came in at 3-1.

'The losers you forget about very quickly,' my man added.

It's the same with drinking. I've had no trouble at all remembering the good times; I've been banging on about them for pages now. As for the other times, that's a different matter. OK, the few really bad episodes, featuring vomiting and all manner of assorted blunders, do stick in the mind because they're shocking. But, on reflection, more shocking to me is the revelation that most of the drinking I've done is entirely forgettable; decidedly, shockingly, boring. Night after night I'd go out for a drink because I couldn't really think of anything else to do.

These nights were overwhelmingly featureless and therefore unmemorable. This was was mindless drinking; not mindless in the sense of standing in the road with a traffic cone on your head singing football songs at two o'clock in the morning, but mindless as in synonyms suggested by my *Chambers Thesaurus*:

mindless / *adjective*
1. thoughtless, senseless, illogical, irrational, stupid, foolish, witless, dull, unintelligent, gratuitous, negligent

Tick, tick, tick, tick, tick etc. And even more appropriate to all my forgotten drinking is the second definition of mindless:

2. mechanical, automatic, robotic, tedious, routine, involuntary, instinctive

These adjectives ring so loud and true that they leave me with a kind of psychological tinnitus.

While the specifics of these boring days and evenings have done nothing to earn places in my memory bank, here are a few examples of the kind of drinking I'm talking about.

● I'd go out after I'd eaten and not really fancy any beer as I was feeling too full, but I'd force it down. I'd sit there, stuffed full of liquid and solids, burping quietly and tasting the night's meal repeating on me. A Geordie friend of mine called this unpleasant condition 'having a bloat on', and advised that it was something to avoid at all costs. He once actually made himself sick to shift some food out of the way in order to make space for the beer. I'd never do that though. No, not a bit of it. I'd drink through it, however uncomfortable I felt. In this way I'd grind through a boring, bloated, pointless night. *Wasted time*: 4 hours. *Pointless drinking*: 4 pints/9 units.

● I'd go to, say, Brighton, to visit my friend at university there. We'd spend the evening in a pub and all would be well. At that point I'd just want to go to bed, but there would always be a clamour to go to a nightclub. I hate nightclubs but, by about midnight, I'd be standing in a queue for entry to an establishment I didn't want to enter to drink beer I didn't want to drink. Inside, I couldn't talk to anyone because of the noise, and neither could I dance, because I'm a hopeless dancer. I'd shout up one lager after another and stand there hating every minute it. *Wasted time*: 3 hours. *Pointless drinking*: 4 pints/9 units.

● Ahead of a West Brom away game, we'd find a pub somewhere. The craic would be good, but instead of sticking to a couple of pints, intoxicated on my exuberance I'd press on and squeeze much more in, probably three more pints. This would cause me to spend most of the match running back and forth to the toilet. *Wasted time*: 2 hours. *Pointless drinking*: 3 pints/7 units.

● If we won, we'd find a pub after the game and squeeze in another three or four pints before getting the train back. And then I'd wake up as we were pulling into Euston, with a dry mouth, full bladder and thick head. *Wasted time*: 2 hours. *Pointless drinking*: 3 pints/7 units.

● I'd meet someone after work who I wasn't that fussed about spending time with, but it was a good excuse for a pint. If the conversation was stilted at first, it would soon liven up. Since he'd bought the first, I'd get the second and the craic would be good, but peaking. My grandad used to tell me to finish a meal feeling as if you could eat a little bit more. That's sound advice with drinking too. It's advice which I too rarely followed for either food or drink. When I should have been on my way home from this type of evening, having had a nice couple of pints, and a good time, I'd be getting into my third drink. He'd have bought that one which meant I was honour bound to get a fourth. He'd then ask if I'd eaten. I'd say I hadn't, so we might as well go for a curry, which we might as well accompany with another couple of lagers. By now conversation would be really waning and I'd be desperate for bed. *Wasted time*: 3 hours. *Pointless drinking*: Well, I enjoyed the first two pints, but the next four pints – the two in the pub and the two in the restaurant – nine units' worth – I could have done without.

● You're at some dinner sitting between people who you find boring, or who find you boring. You are bored, so you just keep drinking the not-very-nice wine out of sheer boredom, to try to ease the boredom. *Hours wasted over the years*: hundreds. *Wine drunk in this way*: hundreds of bottles.

Going back to my day at the races, it strikes me now that there was something else my gambler friend said about betting that is pertinent to drinking: 'The thing most people don't understand about being a successful gambler,' he explained, 'is that it's less about the bets you make, than the bets you don't make. Keeping your money in your pocket and not making the bet is the hardest thing to do, especially when you're here and you're thinking you might as well.'

Over the many years since he said this to me, I've reflected on this many times, but only now do I see its searing relevance to drinking. Being a good drinker is certainly less about what you do drink, than about the alcohol you choose not to put to your lips. Also, the idea of doing something – anything, actually – because you 'might as well' is worth thinking about. 'Might as well' was, for most of my life, a good-enough reason to have a drink. Now, not so much. I ask myself if I want this drink, if I need it and, most importantly, if I'll enjoy it. If at least two of those three apply, I'll probably have that drink. If it's only a case of 'might as well', I probably won't.

That first drink

The first drink is the best. It feels great.

Unfortunately, it may well be a sign that you are, to some extent, addicted to alcohol. It's because your body's been in withdrawal that it feels so good when you feed that need by taking that sip. It's the same with the first shot of caffeine in the morning or the first cigarette.

The feeling is so potent for you that you might even start to experience it in anticipation, before the alcohol has started to take effect physiologically. After all, you have a lifetime invested in the joy you believe it has brought you.

Or it might all be a complete con.

Either way, for me, however or whatever, it feels great.

It feels so great that, logically enough, I soon want to experience that same feeling again. So, I pour another drink. This is nice but doesn't quite have the same effect, and the third even less so. And so on.

The first drink, for me anyway, brings about a significant change in emotional state. I've come to realise that each subsequent drink represents an attempt to replicate that glorious change of state the first drink achieved. This endeavour is futile;

I've laboured in vain, because each drink brings about a smaller change of state.

Understanding this about my drinking is a major reason I've been able to significantly reduce it.

And I'm delighted to say that I still get to enjoy that great first-drink feeling.

Because less is more.

A funny feeling

I had a funny feeling this morning, after a few drinks last night. I drank more than I'm used to these days. It wasn't a very nice feeling. I had a dry mouth and a bit of a headache. I also felt a little queasy. It all felt distantly familiar, like the taste of something I'd not eaten for a long time, like Angel Delight or a gobstopper.

Oh yes, I remembered this feeling. It was a hangover. This pleased me. At last my tolerance to alcohol is waning. Less is definitely more.

Work in progress

So, job done. Or perhaps not. Who's the gaffer now then? Is it me or is it alcohol? If it's all a battle – as the 'battle with the bottle' cliché has it – am I winning or losing? As a moderator, rather than a giver-upper, I'll never get a moment of triumph, a victory parade and an anniversary to celebrate. I think I'm winning; others might not be so sure. Sometimes I'm not quite so sure myself. After all, I will still look forward to any social engagement a good deal less if there's to be no drinking involved, although, in truth, big social nights out that are completely alcohol-free remain a rare thing indeed for me.

And I still don't really know what to do with people who don't drink. If I'm getting to know someone, I don't know where a long, significant conversation with them can happen other than over a drink or two or three. Yes, we could go for a coffee but you can't drink coffee all day and night or you'll never sleep. You can talk over a meal, but that's not going to last all night either. We could walk and talk I suppose; in fact, I'd really enjoy that. But in my world that wouldn't quite work; it would be tricky to organise. Let's say I got talking to an interesting chap at, for example, the football, and it turned out that he occasionally came to the area I live in. 'Great,' I could never imagine saying. 'Let's meet up for a walk.'

I find very light, occasional drinkers tricky in a different way. I mean the kind of people who have 'the occasional glass of wine' or 'a pint every now and then'. This kind of moderation doesn't really compute with me. It's like people who say they have a passing interest in football and 'catch the occasional match on the box' or 'look out' for a particular team's scores. With football, like alcohol, for me it's too big and passionate a thing to merely 'quite enjoy' 'every now and then'. It's like saying you do the odd bit of free diving, or a spot of bare-knuckle fighting on the first Tuesday of the month.

But I still believe I'm winning. The key thing is to be aware that while you can't shake off these hard-wired, long-held attitudes, you can nevertheless recognise their essential absurdity. You can learn how to live alongside them. The secret of winning 'the battle with the bottle', for me, is to stop seeing it as a fight in which you're a combatant. See it instead as a battle raging around you and acknowledge the harm it's doing to those involved, and the damage it will do to you if you get embroiled. Stand aside. Do whatever it takes to knock alcohol off its undeserved pedestal in your life and you'll find a way of drinking a lot less.

This much I've done. I believe I've earned the right to call myself a good drinker.

Afterthoughts

Gratifyingly, the publication of the hardback edition of this book led to a good number of media interviews, and a great many more conversations in the street with people who'd either read the book or heard me banging on about it. All of which taught me a lot more about my subject. Here, in no particular order, are some things I wish had gone into the original book or stuff I wish I'd emphasised more, or less.

● HYDRATION

I read somewhere that the average bloke needs to drink 3.7 litres of water a day. I found this very difficult to do. Or, more accurately, I found it very difficult to do while living my normal life; I was far too busy running for a toilet. However, I did find that, come the evening, I drank a lot less alcohol. An uncomfortable thought occurred to me: could it be that the reason I'd drunk so much alcohol over the years was simply that I was very thirsty? Surely not.

● MINDSET

If you'll pardon the pun, there's a thirst for practical tips on reducing intake. These have their place. Take days off, alternate wine and water in your glass, choose low-alcohol alternatives, and so on. But changing your entire thinking around and about alcohol is, I've concluded, more valuable. Seeing through alcohol for what it is, is critical. And what it is, is a drug. A drug which has its uses but is not the be-all and end-all. It's not the source of all happiness. It's not essential to your life, and if it feels like it is, then something needs to change. The change I made to my mindset boils down to three key points I am happy to share over and over again.

● It's only the first drink that counts; the rest are increasingly vain attempts to recreate the pleasurable feeling that first drink gave you.

● Never stop asking yourself, before you drink, while you drink, after you've been drinking, how many of those drinks you've really enjoyed, wanted or needed.

● Most drinkers do drink moderately and safely – 14 units or less a week. If you drink more than that, perhaps a lot more than that, as I did, then you are among the outliers. If the people you've arranged around you in your life are drinking as much as you are, that changes nothing. It's you and your mates who aren't the norm.

● DRINKERS ARE ADDICTS

I relate in the book how, when I first met Professor Nutt, he called me out for having a glass of red wine in my hand when an hour or so earlier I'd told him in front of a live audience that I didn't take drugs. That evening we also discussed coffee. I said I got a real buzz and sense of wellbeing from my first cup in the morning. He explained that this was because I was, to some extent, addicted to it. Overnight I'd gone into withdrawal from caffeine, therefore taking some in the morning was bound to be pleasurable. But what it amounted to was feeding my addiction.

Two things now strike me about that conversation, pertaining to the 'first drink' point above.

● The pleasurable feeling that the first drink gives me is, I'm afraid, all about addiction. As with coffee, I've been in withdrawal from alcohol so taking some is pleasurable.

● Tellingly, as with alcohol, it's only the first coffee of the day that gives me that buzz.

● **THE WORDS 'ALCOHOLIC' AND 'ALCOHOLISM'**

Clinically, as I understand it, alcoholism isn't a thing any more than 'smokerism' is a thing for smokers. I'm with Lee Mack on this: alcohol is an addictive drug. If you drink regularly, but only a little, you're a bit addicted. If you drink more than that, you're a bit more addicted. If you drink loads, then you're very addicted. If that's the case, then, one way or another, you're going to end up in trouble. And whether or not you resemble the 'alcoholic' stereotype – flushed, vodka for breakfast, waking up in a skip, etc. – is almost beside the point.

At the beginning of almost every interview I've done about the book, I've made my thoughts on this clear. Invariably, the interviewer would nod in understanding. But the idea of alcoholism has deep roots in our thinking; roots that are apparently impossible to pull up. In most cases, within minutes, almost despite themselves, the same interviewer would take a deep breath and ask, *but are you an alcoholic?*

I despair.

To my mind, for a drinker, the key question to ask yourself isn't *if* you are addicted to alcohol. It's *how addicted to alcohol are you?* For me, the honest answer would have been, 'Very'. Now it's, 'Much Less'.

● YOU CAN BECOME ONE

Making alcohol an -ism leads to it being thought of as a disease. And this in turn leads to a potentially fatal misunderstanding. As Susan Laurie, author of *From Rock Bottom To Sober Forever*, puts it: 'I wish people understood that it can take a long time to drink yourself into being a problem drinker. It doesn't just happen.'

This might seem obvious, but it's worth dwelling on. Because I suspect that at some level, if you believe alcoholism is a disease which you have or haven't got, then your assumption might be that this will show itself the moment you take your first sip. And if you're OK after the first couple of drinks then you're in the clear. It's as if this 'disease' of 'alcoholism' is akin to an intolerance of gluten or a serious allergic reaction to nuts: in other words, conditions which, it'll immediately become clear, you either have or haven't got. Alcohol – or alcoholism, if you must – generally isn't like that.

● A GREY AREA

We don't like grey areas; certainties are easier to deal with. Alcohol is rather like Covid, which killed some people, while others didn't know they had it. This made it harder to take seriously. If Covid was like Ebola, which we understand to be always serious and frequently fatal, then lockdown would have enforced itself. As it was, many people saw the mixed picture, fancied their chances, and resolved to ignore the public health advice.

Our attitude to drinking can feel a bit like that.

● NEVILLE SOUTHALL

Big Nev, of Everton and Wales, was one of the greatest goal-keepers in the world. Unusually for a footballer of his vintage, he never touched a drop of alcohol. I doubt this is unrelated to the fact that he was often regarded as a bit of an eccentric. I worked with him recently and asked him what it was like being teetotal in a football environment. He told me how he used to watch his teammates 'rushing around like mad' trying to get a drink after matches before boarding the team bus. 'I always thought, what's that all about?' said Nev. *Rushing around like mad*. Those words rang so true. That was me, always running around, arriving early, leaving late, adjusting my schedule, changing plans, just so I could get a quick drink. As Nev says, what was that all about?

● A SOBER WORLD CUP

As it was held in the dry nation of Qatar, there was very little drinking at the 2022 Football World Cup. In their first game, Saudi Arabia rocked planet football by beating the eventual winners, Argentina. Did we look at the jubilant Saudi fans and think, 'Poor souls, if only they could drink alcohol they could celebrate properly'? Of course not!

If England had won the tournament, their fans at the final would have been ecstatic to have seen Harry Kane lift the famous trophy. Do we think that as those fans filed out of the ground afterwards they would have reflected happily on one of the greatest experiences of their lives? Or lamented that it would have been so much better if they'd been full of beer?

Lesson: alcohol can be all very nice but it is not absolutely key to the experience of joy.

● IN-BETWEEN DRINKING

I've got a friend, a bloke my age, who supports the same team as me. Whenever I bump into him, before or after matches, he has a drink in his hand and plenty more inside him. I saw him recently on a non-match day. I was hosting an event for the supporters' club he runs and he put me up for the night. The event wrapped up before ten o'clock. On the way back to his house I assumed we'd be popping to the pub. 'Pub?' he said, as if this was an extraordinary idea. It turned out that he hardly ever drank alcohol apart from at football matches. I was quite stunned. I had him down as a massive drinker as he drank more than me on match days. But it was me who was the massive drinker, because of all the drinking I was doing not just at matches but on the days in between.

● DRINKERS WE KNOW

All big drinkers can give you countless examples of people who drink more than them. What about examples of those who drink less than them? Not so much.

● THE DESIGNATED DRINKER

A friend told me her problem was that she was the person all her friends would turn to when they wanted to go out drinking: 'They'd say, "Let's go out and get smashed," and I'd say, "Yeah, great, absolutely". It was like I was always the designated drinker. And I'd be letting them down if I didn't deliver.'

'But I loved it,' she conceded. Yes, me too.

● EMLYN THE FARMER

I've just spent a few days working on a hill farm near Dolgellau, in northwest Wales, for a television programme. The farmer and his wife kindly asked me to stay at the farmhouse with them. On the first night, before dinner with them and their children, Emlyn asked me if I wanted a beer. I told him I did, he got us a bottle each, and I settled in for a standard night of drinking, eating and talking. We just drank water with the meal but, settling down in front of the television after dinner, Emlyn handed me another bottle of beer. And those two bottles of beer were all I drank.

Now in my world there would most likely have been more than one beer before the meal, wine with it, and more of either or both sitting in front of the television afterwards. To some extent this would still be my norm. At first I was disappointed by Emlyn's norm, but his norm was better than mine. It was a nice evening, and more alcohol would have improved it not a jot. I'm still working towards making my norm more like Emlyn's.

● WHAT DO YOU REGRET?

Consider how many times in your life you've woken up in the morning and wished that you hadn't drunk quite as much the night before. Then consider how many times, if ever, you've woken up in the morning and said to yourself: 'You know what? I really didn't have enough to drink last night; I wish I'd drunk more.'

Now, what does this tell us? If you often regret doing too much of something and rarely regret doing too little of it, then it makes an awful lot of sense to find a way of doing less of it.

Thanks

Sincere thanks to everyone I've quoted in this book, for their candour and wisdom, or at least one of the two.

Special thanks are due to a couple of key people who aren't mentioned: James Morris, an expert in the stigma associated with alcohol problems. And Claire Garnett, creator of the *Drink Less* app.

In addition to those who are referenced in the book, I must thank the many academics and clinicians who've given me so much of their time sharing their expertise. Among them, Colin Angus, Edward Barrett, James Bowler, Anna Chiles, Jonathan Darby, Matt Field, Sir Ian Gilmore, James Goodwin, Anita Goraya, Phil Hammond, Charlotte Hodgens, Jess Harvey, Lynne Jones and Soren Petter.

Gratitude, as ever, to Hilary Jauncey for being utterly indispensable in every way.

Thanks to Fatima Salaria for commissioning *Drinkers Like Me* for BBC Television. And to Laurence Turnbull, Jess Austin and Jo Ball for being so great to work with when it came to making it.

I'm very grateful to Peter Wall, who describes himself as a recovering alcoholic, for all his good-humoured support. And to his daughter Sarah Wall – a 'clumsy binge-drinker' in her father's view; 'not a vommer' in her own view.

Thanks to everyone at Profile Books, especially Ed Lake and Valentina Zanca for coming to me in the first place, Mark Ellingham for getting me over the line, and Niamh Murray for holding my hand through publication.

And finally thanks to my daughters, Sian and Evie, who all their lives have put with up with my Mum administering neat Croatian brandy to their cuts and bruises; to my Dad and brother Nev for joining us in drinking the stuff, and to Kath for forcing some down with her usual good cheer.